MRCOG

SURVIVAL GUIDE

Second Edition

Khaldoun W Sharif

MBBCh (Hons), MRCOG, MFFP, MD
Consultant Obstetrician and Gynaecologist,
Director of Assisted Conception Services,
Birmingham Women's Hospital,
Birmingham B15 2TG, UK

Judith B Weaver

FRCOG, FRCS, MD
Consultant Obstetrician,
Birmingham Women's Hospital,
Birmingham B15 2TG, UK

Foreword by
John R Newton

MD, FRCOG, MFFP, LLM
Professor
Academic Department of Obstetrics and Gynaecology,
University of Birmingham

 W. B. SAUNDERS COMPANY LTD

EDINBURGH LONDON NEW YORK PHILADELPHIA ST LOUIS SYDNEY TORONTO 2000

W B Saunders
An imprint of Harcourt Publishers Limited

© Harcourt Publishers Limited 2000

⟨ℵ⟩ is a registered trade mark of Harcourt Publishers Limited

The right of Khaldoun W Sharif and Judith B Weaver to be identified as
authors of this work has been asserted by them in accordance with the
Copyright, Designs and Patents Act 1988.

First edition 1994
Second edition 2000

ISBN 0 7020 2545 3

British Library Cataloguing in Publication Data
A catalogue record for this book is available from the British Library.

Library of Congress Cataloging in Publication Data
A catalog record for this book is available from the Library of Congress.

Medical knowledge is constantly changing. As new information becomes
available, changes in treatment, procedures, equipment and the use of
drugs become necessary. The authors and the publishers have, as far as it
is possible, taken care to ensure that the information given in this text is
accurate and up-to-date. However, readers are strongly advised to confirm
that the information, especially with regard to drug usage, complies with
current legislation and standards of practice.

The
publisher's
policy is to use
paper manufactured
from sustainable forests

Printed in China

Contents

Foreword for the MRCOG Survival Guide/2nd Edition

Following the successful first edition of the MRCOG Survival Guide it is a delight to write a foreword for the up-dated and revised second edition.

This book is an essential aid to postgraduate students and should allow them to achieve success in the MRCOG examination. This is even more important now that students from abroad can take the MRCOG without having to work in the UK.

This book provides excellent preparation for the College exam and with many examples of the questions which will be presented in the exam. It will, I think, prove to be of great benefit to all postgraduate students, both in the United Kingdom, and abroad. Wherever possible, this guide should be used in conjunction with attendance at a recognised postgraduate MRCOG Course and structured training to allow the student to achieve their own objectives.

John Newton
Professor of Obstetrics and Gynaecology
University of Birmingham

Preface

We were very gratified at the success of the first edition of the *MRCOG Survival Guide*. This second edition, like the first, is meant for those aspiring to become Members of the Royal College of Obstetricians and Gynaecologists. They have to pass two examinations: the Part 1 and the Part 2 MRCOG. This book provides them with practical tips and pragmatic advice on 'what to do', 'how to do it', 'what not to do' and 'how to avoid it' in order to maximize their chances of success. This advice is needed now much more than ever, with the numerous recent changes in the training requirements and the examination regulations and system. These include shortening the training period, abolishing the elective year requirement, introducing the short answer essays, and replacing the Part 2 clinical and viva with the new oral assessment examination. All the original chapters have been re-written and updated to reflect these changes, and new chapters covering the new examination format have been added. Also, the majority of MRCOG candidates remain from overseas, and we have included a new chapter dealing specifically with their training issues.

The advice given in this book is born out of our experience in training MRCOG candidates over a number of years, both formally in courses and informally – but continuously – in working with our juniors. For us, teaching our junior colleagues remains the most enjoyable part of our work.

We present this book to them and to our patients who, in the final analysis, are the most informative teachers.

Birmingham   K.W.S.
                                                                                             J.B.W.

Acknowledgements

We openly acknowledge the invaluable assistance of the Royal College of Obstetricians and Gynaecologists, and in particular Mr. Roger Jackson, Head of the Examination Department, for kindly providing and permitting publication of the MRCOG regulations and syllabus and data on the examination results.

We would like to thank the editorial staff at Harcourt Publishers for their expert assistance.

Special Contributors

We would like to thank the following colleagues who have provided invaluable contributions to particular chapters (indicated in parentheses) in their special areas of expertise.

Abdullah Issa, FRCOG, *Professor and Head, Department of Obstetrics and Gynaecology, University of Jordan, Amman, Jordan; Chairman of Exam Committee, Arab Board in OBGYN.* (Chapter 8: Overseas Candidates).

Khalid Khan, MRCOG, *Lecturer in Obstetrics and Gynaecology, Birmingham Women's Hospital, Birmingham, UK* (Chapter 14: Literature appraisal).

Prakie Persad, MRCOG, MRCPI, DFFP, MSc *Consultant Obstetrician and Gynaecologist, Director of Postgraduate Training, San Fernando General Hospital, San Fernando, Trinidad* (Chapter 8: Overseas Candidates).

General Plan

The following chapters describe in detail what you need to do in order to become a Member of the Royal College of Obstetricians and Gynaecologists. However, it is appropriate at the beginning to outline these steps in brief.

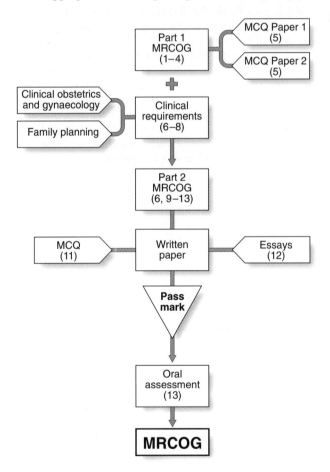

Figure 1: Flowchart of the general plan for the MRCOG (numbers in parentheses indicate the relevant chapters).

You need to possess a recognised medical qualification; to complete a prescribed training programme; and to pass (or obtain exemption from) two examinations: the Part 1 MRCOG, a multiple choice examination in relevant basic sciences; and the Part 2 MRCOG, a written, clinical and oral assessment examination related to clinical practice.

Figure 1 illustrates these steps and indicates (in parentheses) the relevant chapters in the book.

SECTION 1

The Part 1 MRCOG Examination

1

Regulations

Introduction

It is generally accepted that knowledge of basic science is an essential prerequisite to sound clinical practice. The Royal College of Obstetricians and Gynaecologists (RCOG), in line with other Royal Colleges, tests its Membership candidates in basic science subjects related to the specialty. Previously, the MRCOG examination consisted of one part. However, since 1970 the examination has been divided into two parts: a basic science Part 1 and a clinically orientated Part 2. Although several changes have occurred in the format of the Part 1 over the past three decades, the concept of a basic science examination is here to stay. The overall pass rate in the Part 1 examinations from 1995 to 1997 was 37.4% (2209 passed out of 5900 examined).

Eligibility

Candidates are eligible to enter for the Part 1 examination when they have obtained their medical degree. The previous requirement of being registered as a medical practitioner was abolished by the Council of the RCOG in June 1991. In practice, this means that you can sit the examination during your pre-registration training (before 1991 only post-registration doctors could apply). This has a very important implication for candidates. It is well recognized, from analysis of previous Part 1 examination results, that one of the most important factors that determine how well candidates do in the examination is the interval between graduation and sitting the examination; the shorter the interval, the higher the chances of success. By abolishing the registration requirement the RCOG has effectively allowed candidates to sit the Part 1 examination 1 year earlier than previously permitted, thus increasing the chances of success (at least theoretically). The message is clear; start preparing for the Part 1 as soon as possible after graduation.

Overseas candidates

Most overseas candidates pass the Part 1 MRCOG examination at home before they come to the UK, and there are many good reasons for doing this. First, your chances of getting a job in the UK are significantly increased if you already have the Part 1. Secondly, you can never really concentrate on Part 2 preparation with the Part 1 examination hanging over your head. Thirdly, the time you will spend in the UK is usually limited and should not be 'wasted' trying to get the Part 1. Rather, having got the Part 1 at home, you should spend this time acquiring experience on Part 2 MRCOG and beyond.

Dates, closing dates and centres

The Part 1 examination is held twice every year on the first Monday of March and September. The closing dates for receiving the completed application forms are the preceding 1st December for the March examination and the preceding 1st June for the September examination. *Late entries are not accepted.*

The examination is held at centres both in the United Kingdom (UK) and overseas. The UK centres always include London and a combination of other major cities such as Manchester, Glasgow, Belfast and Edinburgh. Overseas centres are more variable and in the past have included Ireland, Egypt, Hong Kong, India, Jordan, Kuwait, Malaysia, Nepal, Saudi Arabia, United Arab Emirates and the West Indies.

Entry requirements and application

Once you have decided that you want to apply for the Part 1, the next step is to write to the Examination Secretary at the RCOG (address given at the end of this chapter). The Examination Department will send you the following:

1. The membership regulation booklet. This contains the application forms, detailed instructions and up-to-date regulations.

2. A list of the dates, centres and fees for your intended examination. The fees are subject to annual review. The 1999 fees are £215 for UK and overseas centres.

The completed application form, together with the following documents, should be returned to the Examination Department no later than the closing date:

1. The original of the Medical Degree or an attested copy. The College will accept copies of certificates attested by the British Embassy, British High Commission, British Consulate, British Council, University issuing medical degree certificate or candidate's own Embassy. If your original certificate is in a language other than English, an attested translated copy should be sent. To avoid confusion candidates must use the *same* surname (preferred or family name) and other names, as shown on their medical degree, in all correspondence with the Examination Department. Candidates wishing to enter under another name other than that shown on the medical degree must also provide their certificate of registration showing the name by which they wish to be registered as a candidate. Candidates who subsequently change their name for whatever reason must immediately inform the College with documentary evidence. A marriage certificate alone is not accepted as evidence of change of name as a medical practitioner.

2. The fees in Sterling (cheque or postal order).

Applications for entry to the examinations held in the British Isles must be made to the Examination Secretary of the College in London. Applications for entry to the examinations held outside the British Isles could be made either to the local organiser or the Examination Secretary of the College in London.

After a few weeks you will receive an acknowledgement of your application and a personal registration number. This number MUST be quoted in any future correspondence with the College.

You must take evidence of identification, which includes your name and photograph (e.g. passport), to all sections of the Part 1 and Part 2 Membership examinations for scrutiny by the invigilators and examiners. Candidates who fail to produce satisfactory identification at the entry to an examination may not be allowed into that examination.

If you withdraw your application for a particular Part 1 examination after the closing date or do not appear you will forfeit the examination fee. Attendance at any part of an examination will count as an attempt.

Two to four weeks before the date of your examination you will receive full details about the examination venue and time, and how to fill the answer sheet.

Pass rates and number of attempts

Currently there is no limit to the number of attempts allowed at the Part 1 examination. When the examination was first introduced in 1970, the number of attempts was also unlimited. However, analysis of the results of the first few examinations showed that the pass rate declined with the increased number of attempts. Candidates sitting the Part 1 examination for the first time had a pass rate of 55%, while those sitting their seventh attempt or over had a pass rate of less than 5%. Therefore, the allowed number of attempts was reduced to six in 1979 and further down to five in 1981.

More recently, analysis of the examination results showed that the pass rate remained fairly constant for all the attempts (Figure 2). Consequently, the Council of the RCOG decided in 1992 to amend the regulations again and allow an unlimited number of attempts.

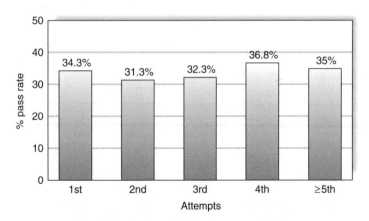

Figure 2: The pass rates in the Part 1 MRCOG Examinations (March and September 1992), broken down by the number of attempts. The overall pass rate was 33.5%. Reproduced with permission of the Examination Department of the Royal College of Obstetricians and Gynaecologists.

Exemption from the Part 1 Examination

Those candidates who have passed certain overseas examinations may be exempted, if they have not previously failed the Part 1 examination. It is worth noting here that withdrawing the application form after the closing date or not attending the examination does not count as an attempt, nor as a failure. It will, however, lead to forfeiting the fees.

These overseas examinations are:

1. Part 1 examination (Obstetrics and Gynaecology), Arab Board for Medical Specialisations.

2. Primary examination for the Fellowship of the College of Obstetricians and Gynaecologists of South Africa, College of Medicine of South Africa.

3. Primary examination, Fellowship of the Medical Council Obstetrics and Gynaecology (FMCOG), Nigeria Medical Council.

4. Part 1 MS (Obstetrics and Gynaecology) examination, Postgraduate Institute of Medicine, University of Colombo, Sri Lanka.

5. Part 1 examination (Obstetrics and Gynaecology), Fellowship of the College of Physicians and Surgeons (FCPS) of Pakistan.

6. Primary examination (Obstetrics and Gynaecology), Fellowship of the West African College of Surgeons (FWACS).

7. Part 1 Clinical MD (Obstetrics and Gynaecology) examination, University of Khartoum, Sudan.

8. Part 1 MD examination, Al Arab Medical University, Libya.

9. Part 1 Master of Obstetrics and Gynaecology examination (UKM/UM), Malaysia.

If you wish to apply for exemption from the Part 1 Membership examination you should submit the original letter (or attested copy) confirming success in one of the above examinations, medical degree certificate and certificate of registration as a medical practitioner (originals or attested copies) and the appropriate exemption fee. The 1999 fees are £215. It is worth noting that these arrangements are subject to regular review and you should contact the College for the latest regulations.

KEY POINTS

- The Part 1 MRCOG examination is held twice every year (March and September) at different centres in the UK and overseas.

- The closing dates for receiving the application forms are 1st December for the March examination and 1st June for the September examination.

- Holding a medical qualification is the only eligibility requirement for the Part 1 examination. Registration as a medical practitioner is no longer required.

- There is no limit to the number of attempts allowed at the Part 1.

- Exemption from the Part 1 may be granted to doctors who have passed certain overseas examinations.

- Overseas candidates are advised to pass the Part 1 examination before they come to the UK for training.

- The overall pass rate in the Part 1 examinations from 1995 to 1997 was 37.4%, which remained fairly constant for all the attempts.

- Statistically speaking, your chances of passing the Part 1 examination are much higher if you take it sooner, rather than later, after graduation.

- The regulations are subject to regular review. Application forms and further information on the latest examination regulations, fees and venues can be obtained from the College website on the worldwide-web on:

www.rcog.org.uk
or by writing to:
Examination Department,
Royal College of Obstetricians and Gynaecologists,
27 Sussex Place,
Regent's Park,
London NW1 4RG, UK

2

Syllabus and Reading

Introduction

The regulations for the Part 1 examination state '…the examination embraces those subjects which form part of the general education of any specialist and particularly those aspects which are applicable to obstetrics and gynaecology'. The Examination Committee of the RCOG has published a syllabus that defines the subjects included in the examination (see below). The phrase 'comprehensive knowledge' is liberally used in the syllabus to describe the depth of knowledge required. The fact that almost 70% of candidates fail the Part 1 examination indicates that the majority either do not understand the scope of the examination or find difficulties in reaching the required standards. In this chapter we will first present the syllabus for the Part 1, then discuss how to achieve the required standards.

Syllabus for the Part 1 Examination

Anatomy

Comprehensive knowledge of the regional anatomy of the pelvis, abdomen, thorax, breast, endocrine glands, hypothalamus, spinothalamic tracts and meninges. Detailed knowledge of relevant bones, joints, muscles, blood vessels, lymphatics, nerve supply and histology. Basic understanding of cell structure.

Embryology

Comprehensive knowledge of gametogenesis and fertilization, of organogenesis and the development of the embryo in all body systems, of the development of placenta, membranes and amniotic fluid and of structural changes in the newborn.

Statistics and Epidemiology
Understanding of commonly used terms and techniques. Interpretation of results of research investigations.

Endocrinology
Comprehensive knowledge of all hormones and humoral agents (both sexes) including their formation from precursors, storage, release, transport, mode and site of action, regulation and distribution in all body compartments as well as their physiological and pathological activities.

Microbiology
Comprehensive knowledge of the characteristics, recognition, prevention, eradication and pathological effects of all commonly encountered bacteria, viruses, Rickettsia, fungi, protozoa, parasites and toxins, including an understanding of the principles of infection control.

Immunology
Comprehensive knowledge of immune mechanism, both cell-mediated and humorally mediated, and of the principles of reproductive immunology, graft–host interaction, immunization, immunosuppression, allergies and anaphylactic reactions.

Pharmacology
Comprehensive knowledge of properties, pharmacodynamics, actions, interactions and hazards of drugs and anaesthetics agents commonly used in the mother, fetus and neonate. Detailed knowledge of the principles of teratogenicity and of prescribing during pregnancy and lactation.

Physiology
Comprehensive knowledge of human physiology with particular reference to the male and female reproductive systems, pregnancy, the fetus and the neonate. Quantitative information about common physiological activities. Understanding of the principles of nutrition, water, electrolyte and acid-base balance and cell biology.

Pathology
Comprehensive knowledge of general pathological principles including general, tissue and cellular responses to trauma, infection, inflammation,

therapeutic intervention (especially by the use of irradiation, cytotoxic drugs and hormones), disturbances in blood flow, loss of body fluids and neoplasia. Detailed knowledge of common pathological conditions.

Genetics

Understanding of the structure and function of chromosomes and genes. Knowledge of the principles of inheritance of chromosomal and genetic disorders. Detailed knowledge of common inherited disorders and of common fetal malformations.

Biochemistry

Comprehensive knowledge of the metabolism of carbohydrates, lipids, proteins and nucleic acids, of the roles of vitamins, minerals and enzymes and of the composition and regulation of intracellular and extracellular fluids. Detailed knowledge of the processes involved in steroidogenesis, placental function and materno–fetal interactions.

Biophysics

Knowledge of the physical principles and biological effects of heat, sound and electromagnetic radiation. Understanding of the principles of laser, electrocardiography, isotopes, X-rays, ultrasound and magnetic resonance imaging.

Reading

The first problem facing prospective Part 1 candidates is deciding on a realistic and suitable reading list. The difficulty is in choosing between relatively small books (with the concern that they may not be adequate for the examination) and large volumes that are difficult to master and know well. Most candidates will be preparing for the examination during busy junior hospital posts that do not lend themselves adequately to memorizing very large volume basic science textbooks. Unfortunately, the luxury of whole weeks and months dedicated solely to studying does not exist after leaving medical school.

Candidates are further confused when some suggested reading lists, which include *Gray's Anatomy*, *Walter and Israel's Pathology* and Topley and Wilson's *Microbiology*, go on to say that these books may not be enough for the Part 1 examination! This cautious attitude, however understandable, is not much help to candidates. Recently, a more realistic and encouraging attitude has been taken by some well-known authors. These authors have stated in the preface of their 298-page book on basic science for the Part 1 MRCOG: '...most knowledge to pass Part 1 MRCOG is in this book...'[1].

A good tip is to start preparing for the Part 1 as soon as possible after graduation. This will ensure that the basic sciences you have studied as an undergraduate are still up-to-date and fresh in your mind (or at least fresher than what they would have been a few years later). We suggest a minimum of 6–9 months for preparation.

Obstetrics and Gynaecology Basic Science Textbooks

Read one of the general basic science textbooks that are specific for obstetrics and gynaecology. These have been written with the Part 1 MRCOG in mind and contain knowledge pertinent to both the content and format of the examination. They also come in small readable sizes.

An important point to note is that these books are *very* condensed. All the knowledge in them (including tables and diagrams) is essential to remember. It is far better to study a small book well rather than a large book badly.

Two basic science textbooks which are particularly popular among the Part 1 candidates are:

- de Swiet M and Chamberlain GVP (1992) *Basic Science in Obstetrics and Gynaecology – A Textbook for MRCOG Part 1*, 2nd edition, Edinburgh: Churchill Livingstone.

- Chard T and Lilford R (1997) *Basic Sciences for Obstetrics and Gynaecology*, 5th edition, London: Springer-Verlag.

These are only two examples and many other books, not mentioned here, are also suitable for studying for the Part 1 examination. You should always use the latest edition of any book.

General Basic Science Textbooks

Having read your obstetrics and gynaecology basic science textbook *well*, you should use the remainder of your preparation time to read general basic science textbooks. Which books to read is generally a matter of personal choice. We recommend the books you have read as an undergraduate (their latest editions) as you will be more familiar with their styles. With regard to what to read in these books, this will depend mainly on two factors. First, you should read about what you have not clearly understood from your main book. Secondly, you should read further about the topics of the syllabus not covered well in your main book. In our experience, anatomy and pathology are two subjects that usually require further reading.

Here we have listed a few examples of suitable textbooks. These are not compulsory and for guidance only. Many other books, not mentioned here, are also suitable for the Part 1 examination.

Anatomy

- McMinn RMH (1994) *Last's Anatomy: Regional and Applied*, 9th edition, Edinburgh: Churchill Livingstone.

- Williams P *et al.* (1995) *Gray's Anatomy*, 38th edition, Edinburgh: Churchill Livingstone.

Biochemistry

- Stryer L (1995) *Biochemistry*, 4th edition, New York: WH Freeman & Co.

- Murray RK *et al.* (1997) *Harper's Biochemistry*, 24th edition, Los Altos, California: Appleton Lange.

Pharmacology

- Laurence DR and Bennett PN (1997) *Clinical Pharmacology*, 8th edition, Edinburgh: Churchill Livingstone.

- Rang HP and Dale MM (1999) *Pharmacology*, 4th edition, Edinburgh: Churchill Livingstone.

Pathology

- Underwood JC (1996) *General and Systemic Pathology*, 2nd edition, Edinburgh: Churchill Livingstone.

- MacSween RN and Whaley K (1992) *Muir's Textbook of Pathology*, 13th edition, London: Edward Arnold.

Immunology

- Roitt IM (1997) *Essential Immunology*, 9th edition, Oxford: Blackwell Scientific Publications.

- Roitt IM, Brostoff J and Male D (1998) *Immunology*, 5th edition, London: Mosby.

Physiology

- Ganong WF (1997) *Review of Medical Physiology*, 18th edition, Los Altos, California:Appleton Lange.

- Chamberlain GVP (1998) *Clinical Physiology in Obstetrics*, 3rd edition, Oxford: Blackwell Scientific Publications.

Embryology

- Moore KL and Persaud TV (1998) *Developing Human*, 6th edition, London: WB Saunders.

- Sadler TW (1995) *Langman's Medical Embryology*, 7th edition, Baltimore: Williams & Wilkins.

Endocrinology

- Speroff L, Glass RH and Kase NG (1999) *Clinical Gynaecology Endocrinology and Infertility*, 6th edition, Baltimore: Williams and Wilkins.

- Yen SS and Jaffe RB (1998) *Reproductive Endocrinology: Physiology, Pathophysiology and Clinical Management*, 4th edition, London: WB Saunders.

Genetics

- Connor JM amd Ferguson-Smith MA (1997) *Essential Medical Genetics*, 5th edition, Oxford: Blackwell Scientific Publications.

- Kingston H (1997) *ABC of Clinical Genetics*, 2nd edition, London: British Medical Association.

Microbiology

- Murray PR *et al.* (1998) *Medical Microbiology*, 3rd edition, St Louis: Mosby.

- Mims CA *et al.* (1998) *Medical Microbiology,* 2nd edition, St Louis: Mosby.

Statistics

- Bland JM (1995) *Introduction to Medical Statistics*, 2nd edition, Oxford: Oxford University Press.

- Faraghes B and Marguerie C (1998) *Essential Statistics for Medical Examinations,* Knustford, Cheshire: Pastest.

Multiple Choice Question Books

Practising **multiple choice questions** (MCQ) should form a major part of your preparation. This is as important as reading textbooks, and will be discussed further in chapter 4. Some MCQ books that are written specifically for the Part 1 examination are:

- Sharif K, Gee H and Whittle MJ (1995) *MRCOG Part 1 MCQs - Basic Science for Obstetrics and Gynaecology*, London: WB Saunders.

- RCOG (1995) *Part 1 MRCOG Examination - Multiple Choice Questions and Answers*, London: RCOG.

- Tindall VR (1992) *Multiple Choice Tutor: Basic Sciences in Obstetrics and Gynaecology* (first +second series), London: Heinmann.

- Chard T and Lilford R (1998) *Basic Sciences for Obstetrics and Gynaecology MCQs*, 2nd edition, London: Springer-Verlag.

- Ireland D (1994) *MRCOG Part 1: MCQ Revision Book*, Knustford, Cheshire: Pastest.

You can also practise by using MCQ books which are written for basic science in general.

KEY POINTS

- The topics covered in the Part 1 MRCOG examination are basic sciences as applied to obstetrics and gynaecology. These include anatomy, physiology, biochemistry, endocrinology, genetics, pathology, microbiology, immunology, pharmacology and statistics.

- Start preparing for the Part 1 examination as soon as possible after graduation.

- It is suggested that you first read a basic science textbook specifically written for obstetrics and gynaecology.

- You should also supplement your knowledge by reading general basic science textbooks. Your undergraduate books are generally recommended.

- Practising MCQ is as important as reading textbooks.

- The books suggested in this chapter have proved very useful for the Part 1 candidates. These are for guidance only, and many other books are also suitable. Remember to read the latest editions.

- A suggested reading list is provided (also for guidance only) at the College's website on www.rcog.org.uk.

---

[1] de Swiet M and Chamberlain GVP (1992). Preface. In: *Basic Science in Obstetrics and Gynaecology – A Textbook for MRCOG Part 1*, 2nd edn. Churchill Livingstone, Edinburgh, pp.v.

3

The Examination System

Introduction

The format of the Part 1 examination has undergone many changes since it was first introduced in 1970. Initially, the examination consisted of an essay paper and a multiple choice question (MCQ) paper. In 1978 the essay paper was abolished and in 1982 another MCQ paper was added. At different stages there were suggestions of adding an oral component, similar to the Primary Examination of the Fellowship of the Royal College of Surgeons (FRCS). For practical reasons, these suggestions were not and are unlikely to be adopted in the foreseeable future. Despite numerous recent changes in the Part 2 examination format, the current Part 1 format has not changed and is set to stay for many years to come. Understanding the examination system will aid intelligent preparation and maximize the chances of success.

The MCQ papers

The examination consists of two MCQ papers, each containing 60 questions (every MCQ has one opening statement followed by five responses – see below). One paper is taken during the morning and the other during the afternoon of the same day. Two hours are allowed for each paper.

The questions in the two papers are divided into sections, each addressing a different topic of the syllabus. The exact arrangement may vary between different examinations, but the following is common:

Paper 1
20 MCQ on anatomy and embryology (18 and 2 respectively)
20 MCQ on endocrinology and statistics (18 and 2 respectively)
20 MCQ on microbiology, pharmacology and immunology

Paper 2
20 MCQ on physiology
20 MCQ on pathology and genetics
20 MCQ on biochemistry and biophysics

It is important to know this information when planning your final revision. As you will see later in this chapter, you do not need to pass in every section in the examination. Provided that your total mark is equal to or above the pass mark, you will pass. A useful tip, if you have limited time for revision before the examination, is to spend more time revising subjects with more questions rather than those with fewer questions.

The MCQ format

Each MCQ in the Part 1 examination consists of an opening statement (stem) followed by five items (branches) identified by the letters A to E. The stem is usually a brief, clear and unambiguous statement addressing an important topic. Each of the items could be either true or false. The questions look like the following example:

1. Adrenaline :
    A. is a vasoconstrictor.
    B. is lipolytic.
    C. increases glucose output from the liver.
    D. is synthesized from noradrenaline.
    E. is excreted as glucoronide conjugate.

In the actual examination you will be provided with a computer answer sheet, a special grade HB pencil and a rubber. The answer sheet contains a row of five boxes for each question and is numbered accordingly. Each box refers to a single item. In each box there are two lozenges labelled **T** (true) and **F** (false). You will be required to indicate whether you knew a particular item to be true or false by blacking out in **bold** either the 'true' or 'false' lozenge. *The whole lozenge should be blacked out.* Other marks like **X** or √ are not recognized by the computer.

You must use only the grade HB pencil provided for completing all parts of the answer sheets. This is essential as the answer sheets are marked by a computer which is programmed to recognize the shade of this pencil mark.

It is important to mark an answer for each branch (by blacking out one lozenge). If you make a mistake and want to change an answer, you should use the provided rubber to erase it. Erasures should be left clean, with no smudges.

A few weeks before the examination date you will receive detailed instructions from the RCOG on how to complete the answer sheet. You are strongly advised to read these instructions thoroughly and acquaint yourself with their details. The examination hall is not the ideal place to be reading answering instructions for the first time. Detailed instructions and sample answer sheet for the MCQ papers in the Part 1 examination are provided in Appendix 3.

The marking system

The answer sheets are marked by computer. Each item correctly answered (whether it is 'true' or 'false') is awarded one mark (+1). For each incorrect answer no marks are awarded or deducted (0).

The marks of the 600 items (2 papers × 60 MCQ × 5 items) are added up by the computer and the total mark is expressed as a percentage. In line with other similar MCQ examinations, the top candidates rarely score more than 75%.

The next step in the marking system is a computer-based detailed analysis of the results to decide the pass mark. This analysis takes into account the general performance of the candidates as well as their performance in specific *marker* questions. These are questions that have been well tried in previous examinations and can discriminate between the weaker and the stronger candidates. Based on this analysis, the Examination Committee then decides on the pass mark. Candidates whose total mark reaches or exceeds this mark will pass, regardless of their performance in individual sections of the papers.

On average, one-third of the candidates will pass (37.4% for 1995–1997). It is, therefore, reasonable to assume that if your total score is among the top third you would stand a good chance of passing. Assuming that the top score is 75% (see above), and that the examination is of average standards (neither too easy nor very difficult), you then have to score over 50%. Some of your answers will invariably be incorrect and you will lose some marks due to the negative marking system. You have, therefore, to aim for at least 60%

presumed total score. This translates into 180 items out of 300 total per paper.

This calculation, as you can see, is based on a series of assumptions. All of them might not be correct for your examination. You should aim to answer as many items correctly as you possibly can. This 60% target score should be your minimum aim when practising MCQ prior to the examination.

The results

Approximately 6 weeks after the examination the results are announced. Your result will be sent to you by first class mail (air mail if your correspondence address is abroad). The list of the successful candidates is available on the College website (from about 18:00h on the day of the results) as well as displayed on the notice board in the College front hall (from 12:00h).

Congratulations are due to successful candidates. Their next step is the Part 2 examination and section 2 in this book should help them through it.

Unsuccessful candidates will undoubtedly be very disappointed. They are to be reminded that many Members of the RCOG have not passed from the first attempt. The Examination Department of the RCOG considers it essential to inform unsuccessful candidates in which topics they have failed. In fact, this was the original reason behind dividing the examination in 1982 into two papers, each containing different sections addressing specific topics. Unsuccessful candidates will also be informed of the grade (borderline or fail) obtained in the sections they have failed. This valuable information should help guide their future preparation.

KEY POINTS

- The Part 1 MRCOG examination consists of two MCQ papers, each containing 60 questions. Two hours are allowed for each paper. The questions are divided into different sections, each addressing a particular topic of the syllabus.

- Each MCQ consists of a stem and five branches. Your answer to each branch is either true 'T' or false 'F'.

- Each item correctly answered (whether it is 'true' or 'false') is awarded one mark (+1). For each incorrect answer, no marks are awarded or deducted (0).

- After detailed analysis of the general performance in the examination as well as the performance in special *marker* questions the pass mark is decided.

- Candidates whose total mark is equal to or above the pass mark will pass, regardless of their performance in individual sections of the papers.

- The results will be announced six weeks after the examination

- Unsuccessful candidates will be informed in which topics of the syllabus they have failed. This information should help them in future preparation.

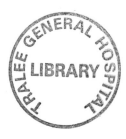

4

Multiple Choice Questions – Techniques

INTRODUCTION

Multiple choice questions (MCQ) are widely used in both undergraduate and postgraduate medical examinations. They provide a reliable and valid method of testing factual information as well as covering a wide range of topics. Furthermore, their computer-marking is totally objective and eliminates any element of examiners' bias. In addition to factual knowledge (which is essential for all examinations), there are certain tips that can improve your performance in MCQ. In the current jargon, these tips are called 'MCQ techniques'. In this chapter we will first describe briefly how MCQ are set and then discuss these 'techniques' in detail.

Setting MCQ

Contrary to the popular belief among candidates, setting MCQ is as difficult as answering them. Some examiners will go even further and claim it is more difficult! The questions are set by a panel of experienced examiners, and are thoroughly scrutinized and re-scrutinized before being included in the examination. Every question should be as clear and brief as possible. It should address an important and common subject relevant to the syllabus. The answer should be factual information which lends itself to the 'true/false' format and could be found in standard textbooks. Debatable issues and mutually exclusive options are avoided. The difficulty in setting MCQ is finding statements that appear plausible but are false. All textbooks mention the true answers and it is far more difficult for examiners to find false statements that do not appear obvious. As setting new MCQ is such a difficult and time consuming task, the RCOG does not publish all previous examination questions and candidates are not allowed to take the examination papers outside the examination hall.

MCQ techniques

Read carefully and understand clearly

Read the question carefully and make sure you understand it. Do not simply *think* you understand it. When you have to go through 300 items in 2 hours it is not uncommon to rush in and misread the questions. 'Adrenaline' could be easily misread as 'noradrenaline', 'oxy-haemoglobin' as 'carboxy-haemoglobin' and 'fetal haemoglobin' as 'fetal blood'. In every question, the opening stem should be read together with each of the options (A–E) and taken as a single item. Each item should be considered independently of the other statements.

Do not read between the lines

Accept the question at face value and do not look for catches or hidden meanings. Trust that the examiners are trying to test your factual knowledge, not to trick you into making mistakes. What you clearly understand from the question is what is meant by it.

To guess or not to guess

After reading (and understanding) each item, your initial response will fall into one of three categories.

First, you may be sure of the answer and have no doubt about the correct response (whether true or false) – go ahead and without hesitation answer the question.

Secondly, there are those items about which you are not quite certain and yet they 'ring a bell'. You may not immediately know the answer, but from your basic knowledge you could reason it out from first principles – go for it and play your hunches. Such educated hunches that are based on sound judgment and reasoning are more often right than wrong, and you are advised to be bold and answer these items accordingly.

Thirdly, you may be totally ignorant of the answer. The usual advice in such situations, with the *negative* marking system used in many MCQ examinations, is not to guess. However, in the Part 1 MRCOG examination this system has been abolished since 1994. There is nothing to be lost by blindly guessing the answers to such items. If you are incorrect you will not lose any marks and if you are correct (50% probability) you will gain. Readers who are preparing for other examinations which still use the negative marking system should not guess blindly.

What is the pass mark?

At the time of your examination no body knows the answer to this question, not even the examiners. As we have seen in the previous chapter, the Part 1 is a norm-referenced examination where the performance of all the candidates has to be analysed before the pass mark is decided. It is, therefore, wrong to assume that there is a 'safe' score, count your responses until you reach it and then stop. You should aim to score as high as possible.

Organize your time

In the Part 1 MRCOG examination you are allowed 2 hours for every paper (60 questions), which translates into 2 minutes per question (5 items) or 24 seconds per item. This might appear too little, but it is not. The items you are sure of will take only a few seconds. The same applies to those items about which you are totally ignorant. We suggest you go through the whole paper first, answering those questions to which you are sure you know the answers. As you are unlikely to change these answers, you are advised to record them on the answer sheet from the outset. The remaining time should be directed to the unanswered, more time-consuming items about which you are uncertain but have enough basic knowledge to make reasoned hunches. You should have marked these items on the question paper during your first reading to facilitate coming back to them. Any remaining time should be spent on revising the answers, but remember that your first thought is likely to be the correct answer.

Fill-in the answer sheet correctly

A sure recipe for disaster in MCQ examinations is to make a systematic error in recording the answers. If you answer question 1 in place of question 2, all the following answers will also be recorded wrongly. Such mistakes are quite easily done under the stress of the examination. Make sure when you fill-in every answer that it is in the right place.

MCQ terminology

Candidates may find difficulty in understanding some words commonly used in MCQ. The following is a guide to the accepted meanings of some of these troublesome words:

- Common/ characteristic/ usual/ typical: what is expected to be found in the average, textbook description.

- Recognized/ may occur/ can occur: has been described, even if rarely.

- Essential feature: must occur to make a diagnosis.

- Frequently/ often: imply a rate of occurrence greater than 50%.

- Never: 0%.

- Always: 100%.

- Rare: < 5%.

Beware that absolutes are very rare in medicine. Items that contain always or never are often false.

Practising MCQ

This is as important as reading textbooks and should form 50% of your preparation. Practising MCQ will familiarize you with the examination system and help identify areas of weakness in your knowledge. Some MCQ books (written specifically for the Part 1 candidates) are listed in Chapter 2. Other basic science MCQ books will also be useful. You should use these for self-assessment (i.e. attempt to answer the questions before looking at the provided answers). The practice and experience you will gain in reasoning and educated hunches will go a long way to maximize your score in the actual examination.

KEY POINTS

- The Part 1 examination questions are clear and brief, address important and common subjects and test factual non-controversial knowledge.

- When answering MCQ, read the stem and each option carefully, understand them clearly and consider them independently of other options.

- Take each question at its face value.

- Work out the answers by educated reasoning from basic principles.

- If you do not know the answer, guess. There is no negative marking system in the Part 1 examination. If you guess an answer there is (at least theoretically) a 50% chance of getting it right, and nothing to loose.

- Aim to score as high as possible and do not assume that there is a safe score above which you do not need to attempt any more questions.

- Mark your answers clearly and accurately and keep an eye on the time.

5

Multiple Choice Questions – Examples

The following 180 questions are similar to the Part 1 questions in both style and content. They are arranged in six 30-question papers. Every two papers taken together could be regarded as a Part 1 examination paper. The answers are provided at the end of this chapter, but before looking them up you are advised to try to answer the questions from your knowledge. Try to practise against the clock, giving 1 hour for each group.

Paper 1 (questions 1–30):

1. The ureter in the adult female:
   A. crosses under the uterine artery.
   B. is ectodermal in origin.
   C. crosses under the genito-femoral nerve.
   D. crosses under the ovarian vessels.
   E. has a retroperitoneal course.

2. The following arteries are derived from the anterior division of the internal iliac artery:
   A. uterine.
   B. ovarian.
   C. lateral sacral.
   D. internal pudendal.
   E. inferior gluteal.

3. The femoral ring:
   A. is the abdominal end of the femoral canal.
   B. has the lacunar ligament as a boundary.
   C. has the femoral artery as a boundary.
   D. has the inguinal ligament as a boundary.
   E. is relatively larger in the male than the female.

4. The lesser sciatic foramen:
   A. transmits the inferior gluteal nerve.
   B. has the sacrospinous ligament as a boundary.
   C. transmits the inferior pudendal nerve.
   D. has the sacrotuberous ligament as a boundary.
   E. transmits the tendon of obturator internus muscle.

5. The long saphenous vein:
   A. lies below the deep fascia.
   B. originates in the lateral end of the dorsal venous arch of the foot.
   C. passes in front of the lateral malleolus.
   D. is joined by the superficial circumflex iliac vein.
   E. is accompanied in the thigh by the saphenous nerve.

6. The following open into the prostatic urethra:
   A. the vas deferens.
   B. the ducts of the bulbo-urethral glands.
   C. the ducts of the seminal vesicles.
   D. the ejaculatory ducts.
   E. the prostatic ductules.

7. The superficial inguinal ring:
   A. transmits the ilio-inguinal nerve.
   B. is an opening in the external oblique aponeurosis.
   C. may transmit an indirect inguinal hernia.
   D. is circular in shape.
   E. may transmit a direct inguinal hernia.

8. The pudendal canal:
   A. is formed by the obturator fascia.
   B. is a continuation of the obturator canal.
   C. transmits the obturator artery.
   D. is situated in the lateral wall of the ischio-rectal fossa.
   E. terminates by opening into the superficial perineal pouch.

9. The following arteries are direct branches of the superior mesenteric artery:
   A. the right colic artery.
   B. the ileo-colic.
   C. the hepatic artery.
   D. the splenic artery.
   E. the middle colic artery.

10. In the femoral triangle:
    A. the femoral vein separates the femoral artery from the adductor longus muscle.
    B. the lateral border is formed by the medial margin of the sartorius muscle.
    C. part of the floor is formed by the psoas and pectineus muscles.
    D. the medial border is formed by the lateral margin of the adductor longus muscle.
    E. the femoral nerve is medial to the femoral artery.

11. Sites of anastomoses between the systemic and portal circulations include:
    A. the anterior abdominal wall.
    B. the bare area of the liver.
    C. the duodeno-jejunal flexure.
    D. the lower end of the oesophagus.
    E. the wall of the anal canal.

12. A femoral hernia:
    A. has the ilio-tibial tract as a covering.
    B. may pass through the obturator canal.
    C. has the femoral septum as a covering.
    D. may ascend in the superficial fascia in front of the inguinal ligament.
    E. has the stretched lacunar ligament as a covering.

13. The rectum:
    A. ends beyond the tip of the coccyx.
    B. has a venous drainage to the systemic circulation.
    C. is suspended by a mesentry in its upper two-thirds.
    D. begins at the level of the first sacral vertebra.
    E. is supplied by the pelvic splanchnic nerves.

14. The amnion:
    A. is surrounded by the chorion.
    B. is derived from the blastocyst.
    C. in a monozygotic twin pregnancy may be separated from its fellow by the chorion.
    D. covers the fetal surface of the placenta.
    E. separates from the decidua in the third stage of labour.

15. In the development of the female genital tract:
   A. the Fallopian tube is derived from the mesonephric duct.
   B. the clitoris is derived from the genital tubercle.
   C. the ovarian ligament is derived from the gubernaculum.
   D. the labium minor is derived from the urogenital fold.
   E. the uterus is derived from the metanephric duct.

16. The following structures are of ectodermal origin:
   A. lens of the eye.
   B. anterior lobe of the pituitary gland.
   C. mammary duct tissue.
   D. adrenal cortex.
   E. amniotic membrane.

17. The following are situated between the layers of the lesser omentum:
   A. left gastric artery.
   B. splenic artery.
   C. bile duct.
   D. portal vein.
   E. right gastro-epiploic artery.

18. The diaphragm:
   A. is supplied by the phrenic nerve on its inferior surface.
   B. has its caval opening opposite the 8th thoracic vertebra.
   C. has its aortic opening opposite the 10th thoracic vertebra.
   D. contracts during forced expiration.
   E. has the aorta, the azygos vein and the thoracic duct passing through its aortic opening.

19. Serum albumin levels were measured in 100 patients with severe pre-eclampsia. The data had a normal (Gaussian) distribution, the mean was 24 g/l and the standard deviation was 4. The following statements are correct:
   A. the variance is 16.
   B. 95% of the values will be between 16 and 32.
   C. the standard error is 0.4.
   D. the true mean is expected to be between 23.2 and 24.8.
   E. it is unlikely that any of the serum albumin values will be 33.

20. In the statistical analysis of any group of numerical observations:
   A. the mean is always less than the mode.
   B. half of the observations are greater than the median.
   C. if the data is skewed to the right, the mean is less than the median.
   D. the mode is the most frequent occurring value.
   E. the variance is equal to the square root of the standard deviation.

21. The action of cortisol includes:
   A. increased lipolysis.
   B. insulin antagonism.
   C. reduced gluconeogenesis.
   D. immunosuppression.
   E. increased sodium excretion.

22. Androgens are produced or secreted in the normal female by:
   A. the ovaries.
   B. the hypothalamus.
   C. the adrenal gland.
   D. adipose tissue.
   E. the pituitary gland.

23. Thyrotrophin (TSH):
   A. increases both the synthesis and secretion of thyroid hormones.
   B. is secreted from the acidophil cells of the anterior pituitary.
   C. its secretion is increased by somatostatin.
   D. binds to a cell membrane receptor in the thyroid gland.
   E. has increased secretion in primary myxoedema.

24 The following hormones in the fetal circulation are predominantly of maternal origin:
   A. thyroxine.
   B. progesterone.
   C. corticotrophin (ACTH).
   D. insulin.
   E. thyrotrophin.

25. Regarding oestrogen production in pregnancy:
   A. the placenta synthesizes oestriol from pregnenolone.
   B. urinary oestriol levels reflect the pattern of plasma oestriol.
   C. the fetal liver hydroxylates DHA sulphate.
   D. the fetal adrenal is involved indirectly in oestriol production.
   E. the normal placenta has an active sulphatase system.

26. Prolactin:
   A. is secreted in response to suckling.
   B. is a polypeptide.
   C. is produced by the acidophil cells of the posterior lobe of the
      pituitary gland.
   D. is under inhibitory control.
   E. closely resembles thyrotropin-releasing hormone (TRH).

27. Luteinising hormone-releasing hormone (LHRH):
   A. is a decapeptide hormone.
   B. releases follicle-stimulating hormone (FSH) as well as LH.
   C. is stored in the posterior pituitary.
   D. is controlled by neurotransmitters.
   E. is secreted continuously.

28. During starvation:
   A. plasma free fatty acids increase.
   B. plasma insulin increases.
   C. plasma reverse tri-iodothyronine increases.
   D. plasma glucagon increases.
   E. liver glycogen falls.

29. The pancreatic islets produce the following hormones:
   A. cholecystokinin.
   B. glucagon.
   C. secretin.
   D. vasoactive intestinal polypeptide (VIP).
   E. insulin.

30. In the regulation of glucose metabolism:
   A. insulin promotes the uptake of glucose by muscle cells.
   B. glucose-6-phosphatase occurs in muscle but not in liver cells.
   C. adrenaline promotes the breakdown of hepatic glycogen.
   D. lactatic acid is the end product of the aerobic metabolism of
      glucose.
   E. insulin is secreted by the delta cells of the islets of Langerhans.

Paper 2 (questions 31–60):

31. Growth hormone secretion:
   A. is from acidophil cells in the anterior pituitary gland.
   B. is inhibited by somatostatin.
   C. is increased by glucose.

D. leads to increased protein synthesis.

E. falls in response to exercise.

32. The following drugs cross the placenta:
    A. aspirin.
    B. warfarin.
    C. heparin.
    D. RU486.
    E. paracetamol.

33. Oxytocin:
    A. is a steroid hormone.
    B. is produced in the anterior lobe of the pituitary gland.
    C. is inactivated by oxytocinase.
    D. has an antidiuretic effect greater than that of antidiuretic hormone.
    E. may be used for induction of labour.

34. Glucose-6-phosphate:
    A. is formed from glucose and adenosine triphosphate (ATP).
    B. is hydrolysed by glucose-6-phosphatase to glucose and inorganic phosphate.
    C. is a 'high energy' phosphate ester.
    D. is transported by the blood from the liver to all body tissues.
    E. is excreted in large amounts by infants suffering from galactosaemia.

35. Glucagon:
    A. is secreted by delta cells of the islets of Langerhans in the pancreas.
    B. is a polypeptide containing 29 amino acids.
    C. can be used in the emergency treatment of hyperglycaemia.
    D. is released in response to exercise.
    E. acts on adipose tissue.

36. Vasopressin:
    A. is synthesized and stored in the posterior lobe of the pituitary gland.
    B. contains nine amino acids.
    C. is released in response to a fall in plasma osmolality.
    D. acts on the renal collecting tubules to reduce their permeability to water.
    E. is an important pressor agent.

37. Aldosterone:
    A. is produced by the fetal adrenal gland.
    B. causes sodium and potassium retention.
    C. is secreted by the zona glomerulosa of the adrenal cortex in response to angiotensin II.
    D. is the only adrenal hormone with mineralocorticoid properties.
    E. increases blood volume.

38. During the climacteric:
    A. oestrogen is the first steroid hormone to become deficient.
    B. FSH levels rise before those of LH.
    C. oestrone is the predominant oestrogen postmenopausally.
    D. testosterone is the main precursor of oestrogen postmenopausally.
    E. prolactin levels fall.

39. Raised levels of serum FSH are found in:
    A. association with the use of the oral contraceptive pill.
    B. postmenopausal women.
    C. association with the use of LHRH analogues.
    D. panhypopituitarism.
    E. pure gonadal dysgenesis.

40. Bromocriptine:
    A. is a derivative of ergot.
    B. causes inhibition of dopaminergic receptors at the pituitary level.
    C. causes raised prolactin levels to return to normal after 24–48 hours of starting the treatment.
    D. is teratogenic if taken during the first trimester.
    E. causes dizziness.

41. Organisms associated with infection of the female urinary tract include:
    A. *Escherichia coli.*
    B. *Mycobacterium tuberculosis.*
    C. *Staphylococcus pyogenes.*
    D. *Proteus mirabilis.*
    E. Döderlein's bacillus.

42. Normally there is no commensal flora in the:
    A. appendix.
    B. external auditory meatus.

    C. trachea.

    D. vagina.

    E. nasal vestibule.

43. Bacterial plasmids:

    A. are associated with genetic transfer by conjugation.

    B. exist as self-replicating extra-chromosomal DNA.

    C. occur only in Gram-negative species.

    D. may be transferred between different genera.

    E. may confer multiple antibiotic resistance.

44. Bacterial flagella:

    A. are the locomotive organs of bacteria.

    B. are associated with transfer of drug resistance.

    C. are characteristic of Gram-positive organisms.

    D. can bring about haemagglutination.

    E. may be responsible for bacteriophages in certain bacteria.

45. Chlamydia differ from viruses in the following respects:

    A. they possess both RNA and DNA.

    B. they multiply by binary fission.

    C. they have ribosomes.

    D. they have cell walls.

    E. they have metabolically active enzymes.

46. The following organisms commonly cause acute meningitis:

    A. *Haemophilus influenzae.*

    B. *Neisseria meningitidis.*

    C. *beta-haemolytic streptococcus.*

    D. *Staphylococcus albus.*

    E. *Diplococcus pneumonia.*

47. Passive immunisation:

    A. is contraindicated during pregnancy.

    B. should not be used in patients with hypogammaglobulinaemia.

    C. may lead to graft-versus-host disease in patients with marrow aplasia.

    D. is the normal mode of protection against infection up to the age of 6 months.

    E. may lead to serum sickness.

48. Immunoglobulin (Ig):
  A. class M (IgM) is transferred across the placenta.
  B. class G (IgG) has a molecular weight of 150 000.
  C. class M (IgM) is produced in primary immune response.
  D. class E (IgE) is responsible for type I allergic reaction.
  E. class G (IgG) in the human newborn is mainly of maternal origin.

49. Neutrophils:
  A. phagocytose bacteria and fungi.
  B. predominate in acute inflammatory conditions.
  C. synthesize transcobalamin III.
  D. have a life span of 12 days.
  E. synthesize antibodies.

50. Characteristically viruses:
  A. derive energy from host cells.
  B. reproduce only within living cells.
  C. are fully organized and infectious through out their life cycle.
  D. grow in mature human erythrocytes from susceptible individuals.
  E. have specific protein which may inhibit host cell DNA synthesis.

51. Side-effects of bleomycin include:
  A. hypothermia.
  B. skin pigmentation.
  C. alopecia.
  D. mucositis.
  E. pulmonary fibrosis which is reduced by oxygen administration.

52. Side-effects of cyclophosphamide include:
  A. haematuria.
  B. peripheral neuropathy.
  C. alopecia.
  D. gonadal damage.
  E. nausea and vomiting.

53. Streptomycin:
  A. has more activity in alkaline urine.
  B. is water-soluble.
  C. is primarily bacteriostatic.
  D. is potentially nephrotoxic.
  E. is eliminated in its conjugated form by the kidney.

54. Morphine:
   A. is not absorbed after oral intake.
   B. causes release of antidiuretic hormone.
   C. is potentiated by neostigmine.
   D. depresses the vomiting centre.
   E. causes miosis.

55. The following drugs are contraindicated in breast-feeding mothers:
   A. lithium carbonate.
   B. warfarin.
   C. propylthiouracil.
   D. penicillamine.
   E. insulin.

56. The uptake of glucose by the erythrocyte:
   A. is an example of facilitated diffusion.
   B. requires hydrolysis of ATP.
   C. is saturable.
   D. is inhibited by ouabain.
   E. is analogous to the uptake of glucose by *Escherichia coli.*

57. Histamine:
   A. causes release of adrenaline from the suprarenal medulla.
   B. causes local vasoconstriction in the skin.
   C. increases gastric acid secretion.
   D. can cause throbbing headache.
   E. is found in mast cell granules.

58. Heparin:
   A. is a mucopolysaccharide.
   B. can lead to thrombocytopaenia.
   C. crosses the placenta.
   D. is contraindicated in breast-feeding mothers.
   E. can lead to bone demineralization.

59. Ethyl alcohol:
   A. acts as a diuretic by inhibiting the secretion of antidiuretic hormone (ADH).
   B. is a central nervous system (CNS) stimulant.
   C. has no calorific value.
   D. excessive intake during pregnancy can lead to fetal intrauterine growth retardation.
   E. enhances the action of sedatives and hypnotics.

60. Congenital abnormalities may be caused by antenatal maternal ingestion of:
    A. warfarin.
    B. phenytoin.
    C. ampicillin.
    D. ethambutol.
    E. ethionamide.

Paper 3 (questions 61–90):

61. The increase in cardiac output in pregnancy:
    A. occurs mainly in the first 20 weeks.
    B. results from an increased stroke volume.
    C. results from an increased pulse rate.
    D. decreases in the last trimester.
    E. is more in physically fit mothers than in those who do not regularly exercise.

62. In a creatinine clearance test where: plasma concentration $= 3.5$ mg/dl, urine concentration $= 0.504$ g/L and urine volume $= 2$ L/24 hours, the following statements are correct:
    A. total amount of creatinine secreted per day $= 1800$ mg.
    B. total amount of creatinine secreted per minute $= 0.7$ mg.
    C. creatinine clearance $= 20$ ml/min.
    D. if the patient was pregnant she would have normal renal function.
    E. the concentration of creatinine in the renal vein would be 3.7 mg/dl.

63. In a patient with the following results: pH $= 7.0$, $PCO_2 = 80$ mmHg, standard bicarbonate $= 25$ mEq/L :
    A. it is likely that she has a metabolic acidosis.
    B. the hydrogen ion concentration would be 0.00009 mmol/L.
    C. the patient would be cyanosed.
    D. the patient could have chronic bronchitis.
    E. the patient could have fibrosing alveolitis.

64. During normal pregnancy:
    A. plasma volume increases by about 40%.
    B. erythrocyte sedimentation rate (ESR) rises.
    C. iron binding capacity falls.

D. venous blood pressure falls.

E. packed cell volume falls.

65. Ventilation:
    A. is increased in hypoxia due to stimulation of the central chemoreceptors.
    B. is increased in respiratory acidosis.
    C. is decreased by the administration of veratrum alkaloid.
    D. is increased in hyperthermia due to stimulation of the peripheral chemoreceptors.
    E. is stimulated by J receptors in the air ways.

66. Angiotensin II:
    A. is a decapeptide.
    B. leads to aldosterone secretion.
    C. concentration rises in the infant from birth to age 1 year.
    D. is a vasoconstrictor agent.
    E. is converted into Angiotensin I in the lungs.

67. 2-3-diphosphoglycerate (2-3-DPG):
    A. shifts the oxygen dissociation curve to the left.
    B. is increased by androgens.
    C. has lower levels in fetal red cells than adult cells.
    D. is produced in Krebs cycle (indirect glycolysis).
    E. levels rise during the first week of life.

68. Normal urodynamic findings in the adult female include:
    A. voiding pressure = 45–70 mmHg.
    B. maximum urine flow rate = 20–40 ml/s.
    C. maximum urethral pressure in the absence of micturition = 50–100 cm H2O.
    D. voiding volume = 200–350 ml.
    E. bladder capacity = 600–750 ml.

69. Colostrum:
    A. contains antibodies to *E. coli.*
    B. has more protein and fat than mature human milk.
    C. has less carbohydrate than cow milk.
    D. contains epidermal growth factors.
    E. contains steroid hormones.

70. Substances essential to the development of the red blood cells include:
   A. folinic acid.
   B. ascorbic acid.
   C. nicotinic acid.
   D. methotrexate.
   E. cyanocobalamine.

71. Iron metabolism in normal adults:
   A. iron is absorbed in the ferric form.
   B. the fetus gets its iron from the mother by passive transport across the placenta.
   C. the earliest effect of iron deficiency anaemia on the erythrocyte is a reduction in the mean corpuscular volume (MCV).
   D. iron deficiency anaemia is a macrocytic anaemia.
   E. iron stores are assessed by measuring serum iron levels.

72. The increase in uterine blood flow in pregnancy is contributed to by:
   A. increased number of uterine arterioles.
   B. increased diameter of placental bed vessels.
   C. reduced arterio-venous resistance in the placenta.
   D. reduced angiotensin II levels.
   E. increased blood volume.

73. Changes in liver function in normal pregnancy include:
   A. an increase in heat stable fraction of serum alkaline phosphatase.
   B. a rise in aspartate aminotransferase.
   C. a rise in serum albumin.
   D. a rise in serum cholesterol.
   E. a fall in total protein concentration.

74. Changes in respiratory function in normal pregnancy include:
   A. an increase in respiratory rate.
   B. an increase in vital capacity.
   C. a reduction in residual volume.
   D. an increase in oxygen consumption.
   E. an increase in minute volume.

75. The heart rate:
   A. is increased in pregnancy.
   B. is increased in hypothermia.
   C. is increased with ritodrine.

D. is normally a reflection of the activity of the sino-atrial node.

E. may be decreased in obstructive jaundice.

76. Disseminated intravascular coagulation:
    A. occurs as a primary phenomenon.
    B. is associated with missed abortion.
    C. may affect myometrial function.
    D. may not be associated with haemorrhage.
    E. can be diagnosed by finding fibrinogen degradation products in plasma.

77. Fetal haemoglobin (Hb F):
    A. has a high oxygen affinity.
    B. contains alpha and beta chains.
    C. shifts the oxygen dissociation curve to the left.
    D. is the only type of haemoglobin present during the intrauterine life.
    E. is resistant to denaturation by strong alkali.

78. In the normal adult human:
    A. the PR interval should not exceed 0.3.
    B. the second heart sound represents aortic and mitral valves closure.
    C. ejection from the left ventricle occurs during the period of isometric contraction phase.
    D. contraction of the atria contributes about one-third of ventricular filling.
    E. ventricular systole precedes ventricular depolarization.

79. Respiratory acidosis may be caused by:
    A. pH fall due to renal failure.
    B. voluntary hyperventilation.
    C. uretero-sigmoid anastomosis.
    D. chronic bronchitis.
    E. excessive sedation.

80. Vasoconstriction in the systemic circulation:
    A. can occur due to chemoreceptor stimulation.
    B. is mediated by the vagus nerve when there is hypotension.
    C. is caused by local accumulation of lactate.
    D. causes a rise in peripheral resistance.
    E. may be caused by the administration of syntometrine.

81. Increased vascular permeability in acute inflammation may be due to:
    A. histamine.
    B. serotonin.
    C. cortisol.
    D. plasma kinins.
    E. globulin permeability factor.

82. The following statements regarding cellular damage are correct:
    A. in hyaline degeneration the cytoplasm is eosinophilic.
    B. hydropic degeneration is irreversible.
    C. pyknosis refers to nuclear shrinkage and clumping of chromatin.
    D. striated muscles may undergo necrosis in acute fevers.
    E. karyorrhexis refers to nuclear digestion.

83. Hormone secreting tumours of the ovary include:
    A. granulosa cell tumour.
    B. Brenner tumour.
    C. arrhenoblastoma.
    D. dysgerminoma.
    E. fibroma.

84. The following are histological features of sarcoidosis:
    A. Schaumann bodies.
    B. Langhan giant cells.
    C. round cell infiltration.
    D. caseation.
    E. epitheloid cells.

85. Cancer ovary:
    A. has an overall 5-year survival rate of 75%.
    B. the omentum is a frequent site for metastases.
    C. pelvic irradiation is a predisposing factor.
    D. histologically is most commonly of germ cell origin.
    E. is more common in women with positive family history.

86. Regarding the effect of ionizing radiation on tissue:
    A. epithelial cells are more sensitive than connective tissue cells.
    B. bones and muscles are relatively radioresistant.
    C. can lead to delayed meiosis.

D. high local oxygen concentration is protective.

E. may cause osteosarcoma.

87. The following conditions are inherited as X-linked recessive:
    A. galactosaemia.
    B. cystic fibrosis.
    C. haemophilia.
    D. Christmas disease.
    E. nephrogenic diabetes insipidus.

88. Phagocytosis is a function of:
    A. neutrophils.
    B. lymphocytes.
    C. histiocytes.
    D. squamous cells.
    E. eosinophil polymorphonuclear leucocytes.

89. Mitochondria:
    A. are found in all prokaryotic cells.
    B. are found in all eukaryotic cells.
    C. contain DNA.
    D. contain ribosomes.
    E. store energy as ATP.

90. The following are endodermal in origin:
    A. the heart.
    B. the spleen.
    C. the adrenal cortex.
    D. the dermis.
    E. the germ cells.

Paper 4 (questions 91–120):

91. The following are tumours which characteristically arise in the ovary:
    A. melanoma.
    B. seminoma.
    C. teratoma.
    D. endometrioid carcinoma.
    E. endodermal sinus tumour.

92. An embolus can be formed of:
   A. tumour cells.
   B. trophoblastic cells.
   C. gas.
   D. amniotic fluid.
   E. silica particles.

93. In the normal adult human heart:
   A. the sino-atrial node is located in the wall of the right atrium.
   B. the atrio-ventricular node is located in the superior wall of the right ventricle.
   C. there is a delay in the conduction of the cardiac impulse at the atrio-ventricular node.
   D. the second heart sound is caused by the closure of the aortic and pulmonary valves.
   E. there is no blood flow from the left atrium into the left ventricle during diastole.

94. Platelets:
   A. have similar counts in adults and normal term infants.
   B. have an intravascular life span of 21–28 days.
   C. are derived from megakaryocytes.
   D. play a significant role in the prevention of haemorrhage from the placental bed at the end of the third stage of labour.
   E. are increased in number postpartum.

95. The following tumours are of embryonic origin:
   A. dermoid cyst.
   B. nephroblastoma.
   C. glioblastoma.
   D. reticulum cell sarcoma.
   E. retinoblatoma.

96. Regarding human cell structure:
   A. ribosomes contain RNA and DNA.
   B. histones are very acidic proteins which bind DNA and are involved in producing higher order structures of chromatin.
   C. nucleolus organizer regions exist on chromosomes 13,14,15, 21 and 22.
   D. nuclear RNA is a precursor of cytoplasmic ribosomal RNA.
   E. each chromosome contains a single separate DNA molecule.

97. Histones:
    A. are the major proteins present in chromatin.
    B. are basic proteins.
    C. are coded in the DNA in multiple copies.
    D. constitute the nuclear receptors for steroid hormones.
    E. are rich in lysine and arginine.

98. The major chemical constituents of gallstones are:
    A. cholesterol.
    B. calcium salts.
    C. uric acid.
    D. bilirubin.
    E. magnesium salts.

99. The first maturation division of the primary oocyte results in:
    A. haploid number of chromosomes.
    B. two cells of equal size.
    C. secondary oocyte and first polar body.
    D. the formation of oogonia.
    E. introduction of new DNA molecules in the cell.

100. Normal seminal fluid analysis:
    A. volume of 2–5 ml.
    B. acidic pH.
    C. does not form a coagulum.
    D. count $\geq$ 20 million sperm/ml.
    E. motility $\geq$ 40%.

101. The following are essential amino acids:
    A. lysine.
    B. valine.
    C. phenylalanine.
    D. leucine.
    E. tyrosine.

102. Beta-oxidation of long-chain fatty acids
    A. occurs in the mitochondrial matrix of the cell.
    B. means that the fatty acid is broken down by removing two carbon atoms at a time.
    C. yields products which can be used to synthesize glucose.
    D. is a preferential energy source during periods of rapid exercise.
    E. produces NADH and $FADH_2$ as sources of ATP production.

103. Glucose transport into the muscle is:
   A. active.
   B. inhibited by cellular energy.
   C. rate limiting to glucose metabolism.
   D. a symport system.
   E. dependent on extracellular sodium.

104. Placental transfer of amino acids:
   A. occurs even when fetal blood levels are higher than maternal.
   B. is a mediated diffusion process.
   C. is not inhibited by anoxia.
   D. is a blood flow-limited process.
   E. is necessary for fetal growth.

105. The urea cycle:
   A. supplies the daily requirement for arginine in the newborn.
   B. converts urea to uric acid.
   C. converts ammonia to urea.
   D. acts as an energy-supplying mechanism.
   E. converts urea to ammonia and carbon dioxide.

106. In carbohydrate metabolism:
   A. glycolysis is the main aerobic metabolic pathway.
   B. excessive carbohydrate intake increases body weight due to increased carbohydrate stores.
   C. complete breakdown of a glucose molecule under normal conditions yields 38 ATP molecules.
   D. adrenaline mobilizes liver and muscle glycogen.
   E. intravenous glucose results in a greater release of insulin than oral intake.

107. Vitamin A (retinol):
   A. is fat soluble.
   B. has limited reserves in the liver.
   C. may be teratogenic in high doses.
   D. is exclusively from plant sources.
   E. is important for night vision.

108. Regarding diagnostic ultrasound scan:
   A. the resolution is directly proportional to the frequency used.
   B. the focal length is directly proportional to the frequency used.
   C. the resolution along the direction of the beam is finer than that across its width.

D. frequencies used are in the range of 1–10 MHz.

E. bowel gas enables clearer imaging of underlying structures.

109. Regarding ionizing radiations:

A. beta particles are negatively charged electrons.

B. gamma rays are generated by the circulating electrons of the atom.

C. megavoltage gamma rays have a more skin damaging effect than conventional X-ray.

D. 1 Gray is equal to 1 Joule per kg.

E. can lead to abnormal mitosis.

110. The plasma levels of the following hormones are increased during normal pregnancy:

A. ACTH.

B. aldosterone.

C. cortisol.

D. prolactin.

E. TSH.

111. The following are actively transferred across the human placenta:

A. glucose.

B. alanine.

C. potassium.

D. calcium.

E. vitamin A.

112. In fat metabolism:

A. digestion and absorption of fat are impaired in the absence of pancreatic enzymes.

B. linoleic and linolenic acids are essential unsaturated fatty acids.

C. 1 gm yields 9 kcal.

D. lipaemia represents an abnormal state of fat absorption.

E. glucose concentration in the blood controls fat metabolism.

113. The following separate maternal and fetal blood in the human placenta:

A. trophoblast.

B. maternal vascular endothelium.

C. fetal vascular endothelium.

D. maternal connective tissue.

E. fetal connective tissue.

114. In the normal fetus and newborn:
A. prostaglandins enhance closure of the ductus arteriosus after birth.
B. there is an increase in the renal blood flow after delivery.
C. the CNS is fully mature at birth.
D. the ductus venosus conveys oxygenated blood before birth.
E. there is high pulmonary vascular resistance before birth.

115. During normal fetal development:
A. the first pharyngeal pouch forms the Eustacian tube.
B. the artery of the fifth pharyngeal arch forms the pulmonary artery.
C. the second pharyngeal pouch forms the superior parathyroid glands.
D. the artery of the third pharyngeal arch forms part of the internal carotid artery.
E. the first pharyngeal arch forms the laryngeal cartilages.

116. In multiple pregnancy:
A. the number of chorionic sacs is always equal to the number of ova fertilized.
B. conjoined twins result from splitting of the germinal disc after the appearance of the primitive streak.
C. a diamniotic placenta is only found in dizygotic twins.
D. the placentas of dizygotic twins may become fused macroscopically.
E. there is high maternal serum alpha-feto protein.

117. Regarding fetal physiology:
A. the pH of fetal blood rises throughout the normal first stage of labour.
B. there is a high pulmonary vascular resistance.
C. the heart starts beating at 22 days after fertilization.
D. the pH of the fetal blood is independent of the maternal blood pH.
E. fetal breathing movements are usually increased in labour.

118. The following statements regarding the term fetus are correct:
A. the suboccipito-bregmatic diameter is 13 cm.
B. the submento-bregmatic diameter is 9.5 cm.
C. the mento-vertical diameter is 13 cm.
D. the occipito-frontal diameter is the presenting diameter in brow presentation.
E. the bitrochanteric diameter is 9 cm.

119. In the fetus:
    A. the coronal suture lies between the two parietal bones.
    B. the umbilical cord normally contains one artery and two veins.
    C. the placental-fetal weight ratio at full term is in the order of 1:6.
    D. entanglement of the umbilical cords is common in twin pregnancy.
    E. the anterior fontanelle is easily felt on vaginal examination when the head is fully flexed.

120. The following are homologous organs in the male and female respectively:
    A. prostate and Skene's duct.
    B. scrotum and labium minor.
    C. Cowper's gland and Bartholin's gland.
    D. corpus spongiosum and vestibular bulb.
    E. gubernaculum of testis and round ligament of ovary.

Paper 5 (questions 121–150):

121. The cervix:
    A. undergoes cyclical changes during the menstrual cycle.
    B. sheds its lining at menstruation.
    C. has a lining of columnar epithelium which changes abruptly into stratified squamous epithelium at the squamo-columnar junction.
    D. has a large number of glands opening on to its vaginal surface.
    E. has a peritoneal covering on the posterior surface of its supravaginal part.

122. The trigon of the bladder:
    A. is the least sensitive part of the bladder.
    B. is derived from endoderm.
    C. is the least distensible part of the bladder.
    D. is darker than the rest of the bladder.
    E. lies between the internal urethral orifice and the ureteric orifices.

123. The inguinal ligament:
    A. is attached to the anterior and posterior superior iliac spines.
    B. is part of the internal oblique muscle.
    C. has the lacunar ligament attached to its medial end.
    D. has the ilio-inguinal nerve inferior to it.
    E. has the femoral sheath deep to it.

124. The superficial perineal pouch in the female:
  A. contains the bulb of the vestibule.
  B. contains branches of the internal pudendal artery.
  C. contains the ischiocavernosus muscles.
  D. contains the external sphincter of the urethra.
  E. lies between the two layers of the urogenital diaphragm.

125. The anal canal:
  A. is lined entirely by mucous columnar epithelium.
  B. is developed entirely from the hind gut.
  C. has a blood supply from the internal pudendal artery.
  D. has a sphincter consisting of smooth muscles.
  E. has lymph vessels which drain to the superficial inguinal lymph nodes.

126. The broad ligament:
  A. has the ovary attached to its posterior surface.
  B. has the Fallopian tube in its upper free border.
  C. has the ovarian artery in its lower attached border.
  D. has the round ligament forming a ridge on its posterior surface.
  E. has the ureter passing forwards in its lower attached border.

127. Fetal haemoglobin (Hb F):
  A. appears in the fetal circulation at 20 weeks gestation.
  B. is found in adult patients with thalassaemia.
  C. is not detected in healthy adults.
  D. comprises about 90% of the haemoglobin in the term newborn.
  E. is detected by the Kleihauer test.

128. Germ cells:
  A. arise in the primitive gut mesentry of the embryo.
  B. multiply by mitotic division.
  C. enter prophase of meiosis I only after puberty in the testis.
  D. replicate the amount of chromosomal DNA at the beginning of mitosis and meiosis.
  E. show marked degeneration in the latter half of fetal life in the gonads of both sexes.

129. Structures arising from Wolffian remnants include:
  A. the epoophoron.
  B. the processus vaginalis.

C. the paraoophoron.

D. the round ligament.

E. Gaertner's duct.

130. During meiosis:

A. there are two replications with one cell division.

B. bivalents are seen during 1st prophase.

C. the two components of the bivalent are attached by their centromere.

D. chiasmata become visible during 1st prophase.

E. one member of each pair of chromosomes moves to the opposite poles of the cell during 1st anaphase.

131. The anterior pituitary gland produces:

A. oxytocin.

B. vasopressin.

C. growth hormone.

D. gonadotrophin-releasing hormone.

E. prolactin.

132. Free (unbound) thyroxine in plasma:

A. is less than 1% of total thyroxine levels.

B. regulates TSH secretion.

C. is free to enter cells and bind to nuclear receptors.

D. is raised in myxoedema.

E. is raised in pregnancy.

133. In the control of pituitary-adrenal function:

A. the stress response overrides the diurnal rhythm.

B. cortisol levels are normally maximal at 08:00 hour.

C. there is negative feedback from 17 hydroxyprogesterone.

D. cortisol binding globulin plays a part.

E. corticotrophin-releasing factor is a glycoprotein.

134. Human chorionic gonadotrophin (hCG):

A. is a glycoprotein.

B. has a sub-unit similar to FSH.

C. reaches a peak level at about 20 weeks gestation.

D. is thought to stimulate fetal testosterone secretion.

E. is produced by syncytiotrophoblast.

135. Oxytocin is:
   A. a lipid hormone.
   B. synthesized in hypothalamic nuclei.
   C. secreted directly from its site of production.
   D. secreted in short bursts in the second stage of labour.
   E. important in the production of uterine contractions in early pregnancy.

136. Adrenal androgens:
   A. are important precursors of oestrogen in postmenopausal women.
   B. are synthesized from cortisol.
   C. secretion is controlled by ACTH.
   D. are important in the onset of puberty.
   E. are secreted by the zona glomerulosa.

137. Regarding immunoglobulin (Ig) in the human fetus and neonate:
   A. maternal IgA is placentally transferred from 32–40 weeks gestation.
   B. IgM is the first Ig to be synthesized in the fetus.
   C. transfer of maternal IgG across the placenta is an active process.
   D. all maternal IgG has been catabolized in a normal infant by 3 weeks of life.
   E. breast milk IgA is absorbed by the infant's small intestine for up to 6 months of life.

138. Bacterial capsules:
   A. act as virulence factors.
   B. may be demonstrated by either positive or negative staining.
   C. are all composed of polysaccharide.
   D. swell with specific antisera.
   E. formation is promoted by serial culture in vitro.

139. Hypersensitivity reactions include:
   A. arthus reaction.
   B. contact dermatitis.
   C. Shick's test.
   D. tuberculin reaction.
   E. Ptyriasis versicolor.

140. Organisms that have an important natural reservoir other than man include:
   A. *Bordetella pertussis.*

B. *Listeria monocytogenes.*
C. *Vibrio para-haemolyticus.*
D. *Neisseria gonorrhoeae.*
E. *Treponema pallidum.*

141. During pregnancy:
   A. the half-life of antibiotics excreted by the kidney may increase.
   B. glomerular filtration rate decreases.
   C. orally administered drugs may be more slowly absorbed.
   D. anti-malaria prophylaxis should not be given.
   E. oral ketocanazole is contraindicated.

142. The incubation period of:
   A. rubella is 14–21 days.
   B. gonorrhoea is 2–5 days.
   C. chickenpox is 14–21 days.
   D. malaria is 10–14 days.
   E. whooping cough is 7–10 days.

143. Human immune-deficiency virus (HIV):
   A. is a member of the herpes group of viruses.
   B. could be transmitted transplacentally.
   C. is inactivated by heating at 56°C for 30 minutes.
   D. is inactivated by nonoxynol-9.
   E. causes hypergammaglobulinaemia.

144. Congenital infection or abnormality could be caused by:
   A. *Treponema pallidum.*
   B. *Toxoplasma gondii.*
   C. *Plasmodium falciparum.*
   D. Cytomegalovirus.
   E. *Salmonella typhi.*

145. Erythromycin:
   A. is a beta-lactam antibiotic.
   B. crosses the placenta to achieve concentration comparable to maternal serum concentration.
   C. is used as a substitute for penicillin in allergic patients.
   D. is a suitable treatment for Legionnaire's disease.
   E. is active against *Mycoplasma hominis.*

146. Organisms commonly sensitive to penicillin include:
   A. *Treponema pallidum.*
   B. Beta-haemolytic streptococcus.
   C. *Chlamydia trachomatis.*
   D. *Staphylococcus aureus.*
   E. *Neisseria meningitidis.*

147. Recognized side-effects of prostaglandins include:
   A. high temperature.
   B. vomiting.
   C. diarrhoea.
   D. bronchodilatation.
   E. uterine rupture.

148. Recognised side-effects of beta-sympathomymetics include:
   A. hyperglycaemia.
   B. hyperkalaemia.
   C. tachycardia.
   D. hypertension.
   E. pulmonary oedema.

149. Progesterone:
   A. stimulates the synthesis of oestrogen receptors.
   B. stimulates the epithelial cells of the Fallopian tubes to secrete mucus.
   C. is thermogenic.
   D. is synthesized in the adrenal medulla.
   E. is used in the treatment of endometrial carcinoma.

150. Regarding cytotoxic drugs:
   A. nitrogen mustard drugs are antimetabolites.
   B. cyclophosphamide is an alkylating agent.
   C. methotrexate is an antimetabolite.
   D. androgens have beneficial effects in some cases of breast cancer.
   E. cisplatin is a vinca alkaloid.

Paper 6 (questions 151–180):

151. In pregnancy:
   A. oxygen consumption increases by 50 ml/min.
   B. PCO_2 falls compared to the non-pregnant state.
   C. the ratio of FEV1/FVC is increased.

   D. residual volume is decreased.

   E. there is increased sensitivity of the respiratory centres to CO_2.

152. In a patient with metabolic acidosis:
   A. hypoventilation may be a cause.
   B. chronic renal failure may be a cause.
   C. the pH is usually greater than 7.4.
   D. aspiration of vomit may be a cause.
   E. hyperventilation may occur.

153. A shift of the oxy-haemoglobin dissociation curve:
   A. to the left increases the affinity of haemoglobin to oxygen.
   B. to the left increases the quantity of oxygen in combination with haemoglobin at P50.
   C. to the right occurs with acidosis.
   D. to the left occurs with increased concentration of 2-3-DPG.
   E. to the right occurs in the fetus.

154. Regarding haemopoiesis in pregnancy:
   A. there is a parallel increase in maternal plasma volume and red cell mass.
   B. maternal iron deficiency will lead to fetal iron deficiency.
   C. the normal daily requirement of folic acid is 300 micrograms.
   D. parentral iron will lead to a quicker response than oral iron in cases of iron deficiency anaemia.
   E. phytates reduce iron absorption from the intestines.

155. Tocolytic agents include:
   A. ritodrine.
   B. indomethacin.
   C. nifedipine.
   D. prostaglandin E2.
   E. oxytocin.

156. The following statements are correct:
   A. the lining cells of the Fallopian tube are non-ciliated.
   B. fertilization takes place in the Fallopian tube.
   C. decidual cells could be found lining the Fallopian tube during pregnancy.
   D. normally the lateral part of the Fallopian tube is in close contact with the ovary.
   E. the peritoneal covering is continuous around the Fallopian tube.

157. The following diseases are commonly made worse by pregnancy:
    A. rheumatoid arthritis.
    B. gout.
    C. migraine.
    D. pulmonary hypertension.
    E. bronchial asthma.

158. The following statements are correct:
    A. serum fibrinogen levels increase in normal pregnancy.
    B. prostacyclin promotes platelet aggregation.
    C. thromboxane causes vasodilatation.
    D. pre-eclampsia may be associated with thrombocytopaenia.
    E. venography is contraindicated in pregnancy.

159. ESR is characteristically low or normal in:
    A. pregnancy.
    B. multiple mylomatosis.
    C. macroglobulinaemia.
    D. rheumatic fever.
    E. defibrinated blood.

160. Ovulation occurs:
    A. before the biphasic rise in temperature.
    B. before the LH surge.
    C. following follicular stimulation by FSH.
    D. in some cases of amenorrhoea.
    E. after disappearance of cervical mucus ferning.

161. Electroencephalogram (EEG) changes during sleep:
    A. are associated with reduced skeletal muscle tone in REM sleep.
    B. have the highest frequency in stage 4 of NREM sleep.
    C. have alpha-like waves in NREM sleep.
    D. have rapid, low voltage waves during dreaming.
    E. are significantly altered in pregnancy.

162. The following conditions have a multifactorial pattern of inheritance:
    A. neural tube defect.
    B. cystic fibrosis.
    C. Peutz's syndrome.

D. tuberose sclerosis.

E. cleft palate.

163. Testicular differentiation:

A. is associated with 46XY karyotype.

B. is never found in 47XXY patients.

C. is seen in H-Y antigen negative patients.

D. occurs before external masculanization of the fetus.

E. does not occur in Down's syndrome.

164. A 46XY individual with a female phenotype:

A. may have streak gonads.

B. can complete the biosynthesis of testosterone.

C. has a raised risk of gonadal malignancy.

D. may be unable to utilize testosterone.

E. results from oestrogen therapy given during pregnancy.

165. Pancreatitis in pregnancy is associated with:

A. alcoholism.

B. pre-eclampsia.

C. ampicillin.

D. thiazide diuretics.

E. occurrence in the first trimester.

166. The following structures are related to the antero-lateral part of the left kidney:

A. stomach.

B. spleen.

C. duodenum.

D. jejunum.

E. splenic vein.

167. The following hormones promote maturation of the breast:

A. growth hormone.

B. parathyroid hormone.

C. thyroid hormone.

D. insulin.

E. cortisol.

168. The following statements regarding the breast are correct:
A. it is mesodermal in origin.
B. it lies within the deep fascia of the chest wall.
C. it is an apocrine gland.
D. thelarche occurs usually between 9 and 12 years of age.
E. the alveoli have a rich nerve supply.

169. Recognized causes for low plasma zinc in adults include:
A. diabetes mellitus.
B. anorexia nervosa.
C. polycystic ovarian disease.
D. burns.
E. nephrotic syndrome.

170. The following are live attenuated vaccines:
A. pertussis vaccine.
B. mumps vaccine.
C. rabies vaccine.
D. hepatitis B vaccine.
E. bacille Calmette – Guérin (BCG).

171. Causes of hypokalaemia include:
A. vomiting.
B. insulin deficiency.
C. beta-adrenergic blocking drugs.
D. aldosteronism.
E. catabolic states.

172. The following changes occur in normal pregnancy:
A. the central venous pressure increases.
B. the systemic vascular resistance decreases.
C. the pulmonary vascular resistance increases.
D. the pulmonary arterial pressure increases.
E. the renal blood flow increases.

173. Drugs which stimulate alpha-adrenergic receptors include:
A. phenoxybenzamine.
B. phentolamine.
C. metaraminol.

D. methoxamine.

E. phenylephrine.

174. The following drugs augment the anticoagulant effect of warfarin:
    A. cimetidine.
    B. ketocanazole.
    C. phenytoin.
    D. rifampicin.
    E. metronidazole.

175. The following drugs are alkylating agents:
    A. methotrexate.
    B. melphalan.
    C. chlorambucil.
    D. cyclophosphamide.
    E. nitrogen mustard.

176. The following increase the risk of having a baby with neural tube defect:
    A. folic acid.
    B. sodium valproate.
    C. family history.
    D. increased maternal age.
    E. heparin.

177. The efficiency of placental transfer increases in the third trimester because:
    A. placental growth becomes faster than fetal growth.
    B. vasculo-syncytial membranes develop.
    C. the surface area available for transport increases.
    D. maternal and fetal blood flows become countercurrent.
    E. the syncytiotrophoblast gets thinner.

178. The following antirhumatic drugs are not contraindicated in breast-feeding mothers:
    A. naproxen.
    B. diclofenac.
    C. mefenamic acid.
    D. flurbiprofen.
    E. ibuprofen.

179. Regarding the use of Doppler ultrasound in obstetrics:
   A. the Doppler-shifted signals from blood vessels are within the audible range.
   B. the normal umbilical artery has a high resistance flow pattern.
   C. the frequencies used are 20–100 MHz.
   D. the pulsatility index is independent of the angle of insonation.
   E. the diastolic frequencies are directly proportional to the peripheral resistance.

180. In nuclear magnetic resonance imaging:
   A. relaxation constants are measured in two planes.
   B. one Tesla equals 10 000 G.
   C. fetal movement during imaging enhances resolution.
   D. fatty tissue produces high intensity signals.
   E. the technique is not contraindicated in pregnancy.

MCQ ANSWERS

The true answers are given below:

Paper 1

1. ADE	18. ABE
2. ADE	19. ACD
3. ABD	20. BD
4. BCDE	21. ABD
5. D	22. ACD
6. DE	23. ADE
7. ABCE	24. B
8. AD	25. BCDE
9. ABE	26. ABD
10. ABC	27. ABD
11. ABDE	28. ACDE
12. CD	29. BDE
13. ABE	30. AC
14. ABCD	
15. BCD	**Paper 2**
16. ABCE	31. ABD
17. ACD	32. ABDE

33. CE
34. AB
35. BDE
36. B
37. CE
38. BCE
39. BE
40. AE
41. ABCD
42. C
43. ABDE
44. BD
45. ABCDE
46. ABE
47. E
48. BCDE
49. ABC
50. ABE
51. BCD
52. ACDE
53. ABD
54. BCE
55. AD
56. AC
57. ACDE
58. ABE
59. ADE
60. ABE

Paper 3
61. ABC
62. BC
63. D
64. ABE
65. BCDE
66. BD
67. BCDE
68. BCDE
69. ACDE
70. ABE

71. C
72. BCE
73. ADE
74. CDE
75. ACDE
76. BCD
77. CE
78. AD
79. DE
80. ADE
81. ABDE
82. ACD
83. ACD
84. ABE
85. BCE
86. ABCE
87. CDE
88. ACE
89. CDE
90. E

Paper 4
91. CDE
92. ABCD
93. ACD
94. ACE
95. ABE
96. CDE
97. ABCE
98. ABD
99. AC
100. ADE
101. ABCD
102. ABE
103. BC
104. AE
105. C
106. CD
107. ACE
108. ACD

109. ADE
110. BCD
111. BD
112. ABCE
113. ACE
114. BDE
115. AD
116. BDE
117. BC
118. BCE
119. C
120. ACDE

Paper 5
121. ACE
122. CE
123. CE
124. ABC
125. CDE
126. ABE
127. ABDE
128. BCD
129. ACE
130. BDE
131. CE
132. ABC
133. AB
134. ABDE
135. BD
136. ACD
137. BC
138. ABD
139. ABD
140. BC
141. CE
142. ABCDE
143. BCDE
144. ABCD

145. CD
146. ABE
147. ABCE
148. ACE
149. BCE
150. BCD

Paper 6
151. ABDE
152. BE
153. AC
154. CE
155. ABC
156. BCD
157. D
158. AD
159. E
160. ACD
161. ACD
162. AD
163. AD
164. ABCD
165. ABCD
166. ABDE
167. ABCDE
168. CD
169. ABDE
170. BE
171. AD
172. BDE
173. CDE
174. ABE
175. BCDE
176. BC
177. BCE
178. BCDE
179. AD
180. ABDE

SECTION 2

The Part 2 MRCOG Examination

6

Regulations

Introduction

Passing the Part 2 examination is the final step towards becoming a Member of the Royal College of Obstetricians and Gynaecologists. Candidates, however, are not allowed to take the examination before fulfilling certain requirements. It is not an uncommon experience for some candidates to apply for eligibility only to discover that they have missed out some requirements and cannot take the examination for another year or so. This situation is totally avoidable by paying particular attention to the regulations. In this chapter we will explain the regulations for the Part 2 examination and point out potential blind spots commonly overlooked by candidates.

Keeping up-to-date

At the beginning of your training you should obtain a copy of the Membership Examination Regulations from the College. These regulations are subject to a continuous review and it is *your* responsibility to remain informed of any changes. This task was made a lot easier in 1993 when the College established a Register of MRCOG Candidates. The purpose of the Register is to maintain contact with candidates to notify them of changes in the examination regulations and keep them informed of the names of their College District Tutors and Regional Advisers. It also provides a list of recent College publications and a calender of forthcoming scientific and educational meetings. The current fee for candidates to register is £30. You are strongly advised to register and make use of this very helpful service. This applies to new candidates as well as those who are re-sitting the examination. This latter group sometimes, wrongly, assumes that the regulations have not changed since their last attempt.

Another way of keeping in touch with the College is through its website (www.rcog.org.uk). This is a very useful source of information about the College in general and the Examination in particular. You can browse and down load the latest regulations, application forms, suggested reading lists and many other items, including the list of successful candidates in the latest Part 1 and Part 2 exams.

Eligibility requirements

Qualification and Registration

Candidates are eligible to enter for the Part 2 examination when they have held for not fewer than 3 years a medical qualification recognized by the General Medical Council (GMC) under Section 19 of the Medical Act 1983 and they have, for not fewer than 2 years, had their names (or been entitled to have their names) entered as fully registered medical practitioners in the Register maintained by the GMC.

The Council of the RCOG may waive this provision for candidates whose degrees do not allow them for entry on the GMC Register. In practice this requirement means that you should have held your medical qualification for at least 3 years. Overseas candidates who hold only limited registration or are not even registered with the GMC need not worry, provided that they fulfil the other requirements.

The Part 1 Examination

Before being allowed to attempt the Part 2 examination candidates should have passed, or obtained exemption from, the Part 1 examination (see Chapter 1). Candidates may, however, make a provisional application to take the Part 2 examination in the expectation that they will pass the Part 1 examination at an earlier date. Candidates must attempt the Part 2 examination on at least one occasion within 10 years of passing the Part 1 examination. Those candidates failing to comply with this regulation will be required to pass the Part 1 examination again.

Post-registration Training

Candidates should have worked for 2 years in recognized posts. One year should have been spent in a resident obstetric appointment and 1 year in a resident gynaecological appointment. One year in a combined post is regarded as equivalent to 6 months obstetrics and 6 months gynaecology. During their training the candidates should have received instruction at no fewer than eight sessions at family planning clinics. This family planning requirement is often forgotten by some candidates who are later surprised when told by the Examination Department that they are not yet eligible for the Part 2 examination.

The training should be completed by the preceding 7th February for the March / May examination or by the preceding 7th August for the September / November examination. Further details of the training requirements are provided in Chapter 7.

Dates and centres

The Part 2 examination is held twice every year. The written paper is held on the Tuesday following the first Monday in March and September at UK centres. These centres have always included London and a combination of other major cities such as Manchester, Glasgow, Belfast and Edinburgh. At the same time, the written paper may also be held at overseas centres which previously have included Ireland, Egypt, Hong Kong, Malaysia, Nepal, Singapore, South Africa, Saudi Arabia, Syria, Oman, United Arab Emirates and the West Indies. However, these overseas centres are variable and candidates wishing to take the examination at an overseas centre should check with the College as early as possible.

The oral assessment examinations are usually held during the second/third week in May and November (for the March and September examinations, respectively). These are held in the UK (London) and occasionally in some overseas centres (e.g. Hong Kong for the 1999 examination).

Application and closing dates

Application for assessment of training for entry to the examination must be made on the appropriate form, obtainable from the Examination Department (or down-loaded from the website). The completed form should be received by the Examination Secretary at the College in London, by the preceding 1st September for the March / May examination or the preceding 1st March for the September / November examination. Each application must be accompanied by:

1. Training certificates: original certificates signed by the Consultant-in-charge or Chairperson of the Division confirming the nature, grade and dates of the appointments held and whether or not the posts are recognized by the College for training for the Membership.

2. Family planning certificate: original certificate confirming that the candidate has attended at least eight sessions at family planning clinics. The certificate must be counter-signed by a Consultant who is a Fellow or a Member of the College if the certifying signature is that of another person.

The College reserves the right to refuse an application to attempt the examination for reasons which the Council of the College in its absolute discretion thinks fit. The College reserves the right not to divulge the reasons for refusing an application.

When the training has been reviewed and accepted, the candidate is informed of acceptance of eligibility and sent an entry form. This should be completed and sent back with the examination fees to reach the College by 1st January for the March / May examination or 1st July for the September / November examination. *Late entries are not accepted.* The fees are subject to annual review. The 1998 fees are £360.

Table 1 illustrates the closing dates for the different components.

Table 1: Closing dates for the Part 2 examination.

Examination	March / May	September / November
Closing dates for:		
Receiving eligibility form	1st September	1st March
Completing training	7th February	7th August
Receiving entry form	1st January	1st July

Number of attempts

Candidates sitting the Part 2 examination are allowed unlimited number of attempts. After failing three times, counselling would be offered by the College Career Adviser. As mentioned earlier, the first attempt should be taken within 10 years of passing the Part 1 examination.

Previously, candidates were allowed only five attempts in a 5-year period. In 1988 this changed to seven attempts in a 5-year period, and in 1992 it was further changed to seven attempts in a 7-year period. The current regulations of unlimited attempts came into effect in 1994. This underlines the fact that the regulations are constantly changing and candidates should remain aware of any recent amendments.

Pass rates

Figure 3 shows the combined pass rates in the Part 2 examinations of March / May and September /November 1992, broken down by the number of times the candidates had attempted the examination. The general pass rate was 37.2%, which remained fairly constant for the first five attempts before dropping. However, the number of candidates taking their 6th/+ attempt were small (N = 38), and this drop in the pass rate could have been a chance finding. The overall pass rate in the Part 2 examinations remains fairly constant; the overall pass rate in the Part 2 examinations from 1995 to 1997 was 39.1% (1226 passed out of 3137 examined).

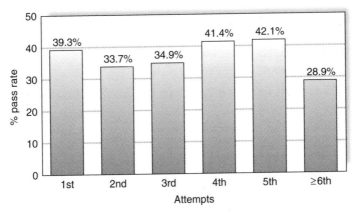

Figure 3: The pass rates in the Part 2 MRCOG Examinations (March / May and September / November 1992), broken down by the number of attempts. The overall pass rate was 37.2%. Reproduced with permission of the Examination Department of the Royal College of Obstetricians and Gynaecologists.

KEY POINTS

- The Part 2 MRCOG examination is held twice every year. The written examination is held in March and September in the UK and overseas centres, and the oral assessment examinations are held in May and November in the UK and occasionally in some overseas centres.

- The closing dates for receiving the eligibility forms are 1st September for the March / May examination and 1st March for the September / November examination.

- The closing dates for receiving the entry forms are 1st January for the March / May examination and 1st July for the September / November examination.

- The training should be completed by 7th February for the March / May examination and 7th August for the September / November examination.

- Candidates are eligible to take the Part 2 examination when their training has been completed and accepted and they have passed or been exempted from the Part 1 examination.

- Candidates are allowed unlimited attempts at the Part 2. The first attempt must be made within 10 years of passing the Part 1.

- The Membership Examination regulations are constantly under review. The College website is a very useful and easy way of finding out the latest regulations. Another way of keeping up-to-date is by joining the MRCOG Candidates Register.

- The overall pass rate in the Part 2 examinations from 1995 to 1997 was 39.1%.

7

Clinical Training for the MRCOG

Training requirements

The Part 2 examination candidates are required to complete a 1-year general training followed by a 2-year programme of post-registration recognized training. This programme includes clinical obstetrics and gynaecology and family planning. In this chapter we will discuss the details of this training programme, and how you should use its different components to prepare for the examination.

General Training

Twelve months residence after qualification in appointments acceptable for pre-registration purposes by the General Medical Council (GMC), or in corresponding appointments in the Commonwealth, or in any resident appointment acceptable to the Examination Committee of the College.

Clinical Obstetrics and Gynaecology

Candidates are required to spend 12 months in a clinical obstetric post and 12 months in a clinical gynaecological post. Each post may consist of a 12-month appointment or two 6-month appointments. Alternatively, the training in clinical obstetrics and gynaecology may be carried out simultaneously in a 'combined' post or posts. One 12-month appointment or two 6-month appointments are regarded as the equivalent of 6 months of obstetrics and 6 months of gynaecology. These posts must be held after registration and the holders must be resident when on duty. A minimum of 6 consecutive months in any one post is required.

Recognized Posts

Only those posts which have been assessed and approved by the Hospital Recognition Committee (HRC) of the RCOG are accepted as part of the training programme. Representatives of the Committee inspect Departments applying for recognition and speak to trainees in confidence. Recognition is not granted until the high standards of practice and training required by the College are met. Furthermore, the Committee arranges 3–5 yearly visits to inspect recognized posts to ensure that the standards are being maintained.

Before applying for any post, you should be sure that it is recognized for training for the MRCOG. In clinical obstetrics and gynaecology posts this is usually mentioned in the job advertisement or job description. If not, you should enquire from the Medical Staffing or the Consultant-in-charge. The Examination Department publishes a list of recognized posts in the UK and overseas, and these should be consulted if in doubt.

Some job advertisements mention that '..recognition is being sought from the College...'. You are advised not to accept such posts unless you have confirmation, in advance, that they will be accepted for training for the MRCOG. On the other hand, if you have started in a recognized post and recognition has been altered while you are in the post, you will not be affected. From 1993, hospitals which have Diploma (DRCOG)-recognized SHO posts as well as combined MRCOG-recognized SHO and Registrar posts are at liberty to place either DRCOG or MRCOG trainees in these posts, on the understanding that posts and timetables will be tailored to ensure that the educational requirements of a particular trainee will be met. Posts occupied for fewer than 6 consecutive months and locum posts are *not* recognized for the MRCOG. Part-time training in recognized posts may be accepted, but approval of the College should be obtained in advance.

Family Planning

During the course of their training candidates are required to receive instructions at no fewer than eight sessions at family planning clinics. Candidates are advised to try and organize these sessions early in their training by contacting their local family planning clinics. Training places in these clinics are limited, and they are competed for by MRCOG candidates as well as GP trainees.

The training sessions could be used towards eligibility for the MRCOG as well as acquiring higher degrees in family planning. Previously these sessions were used as part of the requirements to obtain the Certificate of the Joint Committee of Contraception (JCC). In May 1993 the JCC and its parent organization, the National Association of Family Planning Doctors (NAFPD), were dissolved and replaced by the newly established Faculty of Family Planning and Reproductive Health Care of the RCOG. The Faculty grants Membership (MFFP) and Diploma (DFFP). Interested candidates should contact the Faculty Secretary (at the same address as the RCOG – see Chapter 1) for the relevant regulations prior to the commencement of their training sessions.

In-training preparation

The Part 2 MRCOG is a clinically-orientated examination, and only competent clinicians will pass. This competence can only be acquired through clinical training, which is the most important part of your preparation for the examination. Any amount of knowledge, however great, will not compensate for clinical deficiencies. Candidates who discharge their clinical duties adequately and pay attention to details in their work are those who pass with flying colours. This is simply because the main bulk of the subject matter of the examination is covered by your day-to-day clinical work. In fact, there are many areas in the subject matter that can only be learnt properly through clinical work. Examiners can easily spot the 'bookish' answer from that which is based on clinical experience.

In this following section we will first describe the general principles you should apply during your clinical work in order to maximize your educational benefit. Following that we will give examples of how to apply these principles in some of the clinical settings you are likely to be involved in during your training.

General principles

Engage Mind Before Hand

Always think of what you are going to do before you do it. This might appear as if it is stating the obvious, but it is amazing how many candidates (and doctors in general) carry out routine tasks just because they are 'routine'. This thinking process will stimulate you to understand the rationale behind your actions, which is the only way of knowing if they are correct or not.

Always Ask Why

This is a variant of the previous principle, and applies mainly to investigations. Whether the investigation is simple (as blood count) or sophisticated (as magnetic resonance imaging) you should always know why you are doing it; if the results will not alter the management of the patient then think again. A questioning mind coupled with analytical thinking will go a long way to make you a better doctor and a successful candidate. In the Part 2 examination you are invariably presented with clinical problems and asked how you will manage them. For every investigation you mention you will be asked why. Your examiner may now be a manager within the 'new' style Health Service, and as such is even more likely to ask 'why'?

What You Do Not Know, Find Out

During your basic training you will be faced with many clinical conditions you do not fully understand. This is perfectly normal, and your seniors will help and guide you through such situations. Nevertheless, you should go and read about these conditions after you have seen them so, next time round, you will know more about them. You are advised to keep a small notebook in your white coat pocket and write down the new conditions as you see them. On a regular basis – either daily or weekly – you should look up these conditions in your textbooks. This will give your theoretical knowledge a practical dimension and a sense of immediacy. It will also give you what it takes to pass the examination; a clinically-orientated, experience-based factual knowledge.

Teach As You Learn

Teaching is one of the best methods of learning. By teaching others you will constantly remind yourself of the skills and factual knowledge you have acquired and you will repeatedly go over every conceivable detail you might be asked about in the examination. With the high turnover of student midwives and nurses, medical students and junior doctors, there is no shortage of your potential students. They will benefit and you will benefit.

Learn From Everyone

Do not be too proud and think that there are patients or colleagues from whom you are too knowledgeable to learn. Every patient has some feature from which you can learn. Similarly, all you colleagues (midwives, nurses and doctors) have something to teach you if you are willing.

Do Not Clock-Watch

Medicine is not a 9 to 5 job, especially during the clinical training years. To get the ultimate benefit from your training, you should expect to come in early and go home late. This extra time may not be necessary for you to complete your clinical tasks, but will enable you to gain more in-depth experience.

You can, and should, apply these principles to every component of your clinical work. In the following sections there are examples of how they could be applied in practice.

Antenatal clinics

This is an area that exemplifies the idea of in-training preparation very well. All pregnant women should have antenatal care. This care becomes a 'routine', and consequently some doctors tend to give it without much thinking of the rationale behind it. One of the common questions in the examination is 'what are the routine investigations performed at the booking clinic'? It is surprising how many candidates answer this question inadequately, which is totally inexcusable because it can only mean that they have not been thinking during their work in the antenatal clinics. It also means that they have not been communicating with their patients. For every examination, investigation or screening test you do or request in the antenatal clinic, you should ask yourself 'why'? Your senior colleagues should be able to answer your questions.

Another important and very useful source of information is the antenatal clinic leaflets. These leaflets will not only explain aspects of antenatal care to you, but more importantly guide you on how to explain them clearly to the pregnant women. In fact, work in the antenatal clinic is the only way of learning properly about antenatal counselling, which is another very common question in the examination.

Labour ward

Every pregnant woman has to go through the labour ward (whether for a Caesarean section or a vaginal delivery), and every MRCOG candidate is asked about labour ward work. Here again you should think of what you are doing, why you are doing it and how. As this is a very practical area, Examiners will expect you to say what you have been doing in your daily work and will accept it as long as you can reasonably justify it.

During your labour ward work you should make an effort to learn about, understand and occasionally conduct the tasks that are usually conducted by midwives, such as admission procedures, normal delivery and postnatal care. These are very important tasks and the fact that you do not do them yourself is just a logistic division of duties. You should be able to perform them properly and will be expected to know them well in the examination.

Pregnant women are not served only by midwives and obstetricians, but also anaesthetists and neonatologists. You will work closely with these two specialties on the labour ward, and you can learn through this work more than what you can learn by reading textbooks. Questions about how to resuscitate a newborn or how to prevent Mendelson's syndrome are very common questions in the examination. If asked nicely, your friendly anaesthetist and neonatologist on the labour ward are usually willing to explain their work to you and show you how it is done. This will give your answers in the examination a practical edge, something very much appreciated by the Examiners.

Ward rounds

Ward rounds provide a very good venue for practice for the oral assessment examination. Whenever you are doing a ward round with the medical students, nurses, midwives or your junior colleagues, you should always make a positive effort to explain to them about the cases you are seeing. You should give them a brief theoretical background information, outline the salient points in the clinical history and the relevance of the investigations, demonstrate the clinical examination and discuss the plan of management.

You should also remember that the most important person on the round is the patient herself. She should be made to feel at ease and that she is at the centre of every thing you say or do by her bedside. She should feel that you care about her as an individual with a medical problem, not just as a medical problem. The 'fibroids in room 2' is not the correct name for 'Mrs Smith in room 2, who is complaining of heavy periods due to uterine fibroids'. This patient-centred attitude can be learnt only through self-training at ward rounds, and is very much appreciated by Examiners, particularly at the role-play stations in the oral assessment examination. In fact, it is equally important to maintain this attitude as you ascend up the career ladder after passing your examination. Unfortunately, it is very easy to slip into a self-congratulatory, inward-looking approach to your patients and forget that you should be using the ward round to boost their morale, not your own.

Ward rounds with your consultants and other seniors colleagues should give you the chance to practice your presentation skills. You should always aim for a polished performance. You should also accept and indeed ask for criticism so you can identify and correct your mistakes.

Gynaecological clinics

These present a situation very similar to some stations in the oral assessment examination. The only difference is that in the examination you have to present the case to the Examiners and justify your proposed management. You should apply the same analytical thinking process mentioned earlier to every thing you do in the clinic. Moreover, you should arrange with one of your colleagues, preferably a senior one, to formally present and discuss cases seen in the clinic on a regular basis.

Discharge summaries and letters

These are usually viewed by junior doctors as a boring service commitment with no educational content. They are definitely mistaken. When you write (or more often dictate) these letters you are actually practising your grammar, medical vocabulary and scientific English language which are essential components of your preparation for the essay questions. Furthermore, you have a professional user of the English language to correct them; the medical secretary. They may not admit it, but many doctors have their letters 'edited' grammatically by their secretaries. When you start any new job, you should speak nicely to your medical secretary and ask her to point out any mistakes in your letters. You will be amazed!

Operating theatre

Here again you should have an inquiring mind. Why are we using a particular incision or suture material? Why are we leaving a drain and how long should it stay in? Should we remove the ovaries and why? What are the potential complications? Most importantly, why is the patient having the operation instead of a medical or conservative treatment? Having found the answers to these questions you should explain them to your junior colleagues. This will keep them fresh in your mind and identify any gaps in your knowledge.

Meetings

Many departments have regular perinatal mortality and morbidity meetings. In addition, others have journal clubs, pathology, Caesarean section and

CTG meetings. Generally speaking, there are two types of people that come to these meetings: attendants and participants. Attendants do not prepare for the meeting in advance, come to listen to others talking, and if some of them do not attend, the meeting will go on regardless. Participants, on the other hand, prepare for the meeting in advance, participate in the presentation and /or the discussion and are very important for the success of the meeting. You should endeavour to be a participant in those meetings as this will give you valuable practice in communicating your thoughts to others, which is what you are required to do in the oral assessment examinations. Good communicators do very well in the examination.

Special clinics

If your hospital runs special clinics (such as urodynamics, colposcopy, amniocentesis or assisted conception), you should attend some of their sessions, if only to understand the basic principles. Seeing these techniques in practice is far more educating than just reading about them.

KEY POINTS

- Candidates are required to spend 12 months in recognized obstetric training and 12 months in recognized gynaecological training. These posts must be held after registration, and the holder must be resident when on duty.

- During the course of their training, candidates are required to receive instructions at no fewer than eight sessions at family planning clinics.

- Clinical competence is needed to pass the MRCOG, and theoretical knowledge, however great, will not compensate for clinical deficiencies.

- The only way to acquire clinical competence is through hard work, dedication and paying attention to details in your clinical work.

- The main bulk of the subject matter of the examination is covered by your day-to-day clinical duties.

- An inquiring mind, analytical thinking and a commitment to learning as well as teaching are very important attributes of both a good clinician and a successful candidate.

8

MRCOG Training and the Overseas Candidate

With special contributions from Mr. Prakie Persad, MRCOG, and Professor Abdullah Issa, FRCOG.

Introduction

The Royal College of Obstetricians and Gynaecologists has a world-wide recognition and respect, and its Membership is sought by many overseas doctors. This is reflected in the fact that, at the beginning of 1998, 55% of Fellow and Members of the RCOG were resident and practising outside the UK. This trend is likely to continue as evident from the results of recent MRCOG examinations. For example, in the September / November 1998 Part 2 examination, 69% of the successful candidates had obtained their primary medical qualifications outside the British Isles. Overseas candidates have certain issues relating to their training, and these will be discussed in this chapter.

Plan ahead

Most overseas doctors who attempt the MRCOG are aware at the beginning of their training at home that they are working towards that goal. The course of the overseas doctor therefore goes through definite stages as follows:

1. Training at home in obstetrics and gynaecology.

2. Spending time in the UK before passing the MRCOG.

3. Post-MRCOG experience in the UK.

4. Returning home to work as a specialist.

It is important to realize that the final goal is to function as a competent specialist in your own community, contributing to the improvement of health care there in general and in the raising of the standard of obstetrics and gynaecology in particular.

Overseas preparation

There is no doubt that you should always approach your training as it pertains to becoming an independent specialist in obstetrics and gynaecology. The MRCOG examination (or any other, for that matter) is simply a stepping stone along the way to achieving that final goal. At the same time, however, you cannot get away from the fact that the examination you are going to sit is based on British practice and this must be acknowledged and catered for from early on in one's training.

Medicine in general, and obstetrics and gynaecology in particular, are practical endeavours. As such, you must see and do as much as possible in the early years of your training. In this regard training overseas has many advantages. Some trainees in Britain complain of the lack of surgical experience, particularly in the early part of their training. This is seldom a problem for overseas doctors 'at home' and is a good reason for spending at least 2 years of obstetrics and gynaecology experience at home before travelling to the UK.

However, training without supervision is like going to sea without a map; you may get there eventually but there may be unnecessary voyages along the way. Therefore it is important that you seek adequate supervision. Also, try to discuss the cases you are involved with at home with your seniors. There is seldom only one way of approaching a problem. Learn to ask the question 'what are the options in the ideal setting?' Go to the library and look these up yourself. For instance a patient may be having a hysterectomy for menorrhagia. It is important to realize that the options may include medical therapy, local destruction of the endometrium and laparoscopic-assisted hysterectomy. However, it is equally important to know that there are strict indications and drawbacks for each of these and that abdominal hysterectomy is still by far the most common surgical treatment of menorrhagia in the UK. If your patient has 20-week-size fibroids, a condition commonly seen in the developing world and seldom in the developed, she would not be a candidate for minimal access surgery anyway.

Although a Log Book is no longer required by the College, it is prudent to keep some record of your practical experience. This serves to remind both yourself and your seniors of what remains to be done. It also helps in your job application and interviews in the UK later when you can actually say how many forceps deliveries or Caesarean sections you have performed.

Part of the preparation for your entry into the UK must be making yourself marketable. Remember that when you apply for a job, you are just one of many applicants unknown to the hospital short-listing you. You can distinguish yourself from the other applicants by having experience that others do not possess. Research experience in your own hospital not only allows you to stand out from the crowd, but also demonstrates a deeper commitment to the speciality.

RCOG recognition of overseas training

Overseas candidates should contact the Examination Department as early as possible and provide details of their training. After considering these details, obtaining references from the Consultants, and consulting with the Chairpersons of the local RCOG Representative Committees, the Examination Department will inform candidates if their overseas training will count towards the Part 2 examination. There are certain training posts (in approximately 35 overseas countries) which have been assessed and recognized by the HRC. Some of these posts have full recognition, while others have partial recognition only (i.e. recognition is given provided that a certain part of the candidate's training is carried out in recognized posts in the UK). Early communication with the Examination Department is essential to clarify these points.

Originally, almost all overseas candidates had to work for at least 6 months in a recognized training post in the UK before being allowed to sit the Part 2 examination. However, in November 1997, the RCOG Council agreed that for those candidates completing all their training requirements in overseas posts it was no longer compulsory to work in the UK before sitting the Part 2 exam. Nevertheless, it should be remembered that the MRCOG examination is primarily a test of a candidate's knowledge of obstetrics and gynaecology as they are practised in the UK. Overseas practice and training may differ from those in the UK, particularly with regard to the gynaecology case mix. Overseas candidates should take every opportunity to ensure that they acquire adequate experience in areas of the specialty in which they may be deficient. Practically speaking this means that, as an overseas candidate, you will considerably increase your chances of passing the Part 2 examination if you work in a training post in the UK. For those candidates who have done all their recognized training outside the UK, it is advisable that they spend at least 1–2 months in a clinical attachment in a UK hospital. This will not be as useful as a proper training job, but is definitely better than no UK experience at all.

UK training

Many overseas doctors reach the UK with enough practical experience. What needs to be concentrated upon is the way the speciality is practised in another culture. Remember, the principles of medicine never change; what varies is the way it is administered. This simple concept is fundamental to a successful career in the UK for any overseas doctor. Do not waste effort complaining of the way things are done; simply accept that you are in a different system and adapt. The earlier this is done, the sooner you will arrive at your primary destination – success in the MRCOG. Overseas doctors who seem to have an easy passage through the British system (and there are many examples of these) do not ignore the differences in the way the speciality is practised, but rather acknowledge and accept these.

Leave is available to attend courses, usually 2 weeks every 6 months. You should take advantage of this. Identify courses relevant to the examination early and discuss this with the postgraduate tutor in your hospital. Early application usually means guaranteed approval. Those who wait until the eleventh hour often find that too many people are going on leave and often funds for study leave have been exhausted.

Medical registration in the UK

Before working in medical posts in the UK candidates must be registered with the GMC. The registration regulations are subject to periodic review, and candidates are strongly advised to contact the GMC before planning any training in the UK (address given at the end of this chapter).

Generally speaking, overseas candidates fall into one of two main categories according to their medical qualifications. *First*, some candidates hold qualifications recognized by the GMC for registration (e.g. European citizens who hold European medical qualifications). These can apply directly for training posts in response to advertisements in the medical press (*British Medical Journal* and *Lancet*). Suitable candidates are short listed and called for interviews. Appointments are made on the basis of personal and professional merits, references and, invariably, performance at the interview. *Second*, many overseas candidates hold medical qualifications that are registrable, but not fully recognized by the GMC. There are two ways open to these candidates to obtain registration and training in the UK: to sit the Professional Linguistic and Assessments Board (PLAB) test or to apply for exemption from PLAB.

During 1992, 2380 overseas qualified doctors (in all disciplines) were granted limited registration for the first time (as opposed to renewals) by the GMC. Twenty-five per cent of them held recognized primary or higher medical qualifications, 27% passed the PLAB test and 48% were exempted from PLAB.

PLAB test

Since 1974, the majority of overseas qualified doctors wishing to practice medicine in the UK have had to pass or gain exemption from a test of linguistic ability and professional knowledge and competence before they can do so. This test was originally called the TRAB test because it was run by the Temporary Registration Assessment Board. When temporary registration was replaced by limited registration under the provisions of the Medical Act 1978, the test became known as the PLAB test as it was (and still is) run by the Professional and Linguistic Assessment Board.

Level of the PLAB Test

The standard required to pass the test is defined by the Board in the following terms: 'A candidate's command of the English language and professional knowledge and skill must be shown to be sufficient for him or her to undertake, safely, employment at first year Senior House Officer level in a British hospital'.

Qualifications and Experience Needed

Admission to the PLAB test is open to doctors whose primary medical qualifications are accepted by the GMC for the purpose of limited registration. These include primary medical qualifications listed in the World Directory of Medical Schools, which is published by the World Health Organization.

Evidence of Medical Qualification

You will not be asked to provide proof of your qualification at the time of applying for admission to the PLAB test. However, before granting limited registration to doctors who have passed the test, the GMC will require applicants to provide clear evidence that they hold an acceptable primary medical qualification.

Before entering the test, doctors will be expected to have completed, in countries outside the UK, a minimum of 12 months' postgraduate clinical experience. This experience should be acquired in teaching hospitals or other hospitals which have been approved for internship training by the medical registration authorities in the countries concerned.

A doctor who has not completed such experience may be allowed by the GMC to enter the PLAB test. However, since the test is set at the level of a Senior House Officer (SHO) in the NHS, doctors without at least 1 year's experience of clinical practice are likely to be at a disadvantage. Doctors falling in this category who pass the test will initially be granted limited registration only for employment at the grade of House Officer (HO), which is the NHS grade occupied by new medical graduates. After an appropriate period of satisfactory service as a HO (between 3 and 12 months), the doctor would be able to apply for registration in respect of posts at a higher grade. The time spent as a HO would be counted towards the total period of 5 years which the law permits for practice under limited registration.

Doctors who are making their first application for admission to the test must provide a valid test report form from an International English Language Testing System (IELTS) centre. Applicants cannot be processed until the GMC receives the IELTS test report form.

Components of the PLAB Test

The PLAB Test consists of two parts. Candidates must pass Part 1 before applying for Part 2:

Part I

This is held at a number of locations within the UK. In partnership with the British Council, it is also held in some overseas centres such as Bangladesh (Dhaka), India (Calcutta, Chennai, Delhi, Mumbai) and Pakistan (Islamabad and Karachi). The 1999 fees for taking the Part 1 were £265 (UK or overseas).

There are three medical written papers in Part 1:

* *Multiple Choice Question Examination*
  This examination tests factual professional knowledge. It lasts for 90 minutes and consists of 60 MCQ. There are questions in surgery, obstetrics and gynaecology, and medicine including other specialist disciplines such as paediatrics, psychiatry, public health medicine and

dermatology. Each question consists of one stem and five branches. Each branch relating to the stem could be either true or false. The negative marking system is used here (which is different from the MCQ examinations of the MRCOG) and hence there is a 'do not know' option in the answer sheet.

- *Photographic Material Examination*
  This examination lasts for 50 minutes. It is designed to assess a candidate's knowledge by means of 20 photographs depicting various different clinical conditions covering the three main branches of medical practice. The photographs will include clinical conditions, investigations including X-rays and ECGs, and clinical pathological material including blood films and operation and post-mortem specimens. Four numbered photographs, or pairs of photographs, are displayed on each page of the question book. Candidates will be required, in a separate answer book, to give brief answers to up to five written questions on each photograph. Questions will be directed both to the condition displayed and also to the diagnosis and treatment.

- *Clinical Problem Solving Examination*
  This examination covers the main branches of medicine, i.e. medicine, surgery, obstetrics and gynaecology, and related disciplines. It is designed to assess the candidate's ability to apply professional knowledge to a variety of clinical situations, to interpret symptoms, signs and investigations, and to give instructions for the care and treatment of patients. The examination lasts for 45 minutes and consists of five problems, all of which must be attempted by the candidate.

Part 2: Objective Structured Clinical Examination (OSCE)
This is held only in the UK, and the 1999 fees for taking the exam were £150. The aim of the OSCE is to test your clinical and communication skills. It is designed so that an examiner can observe you putting these skills into practice. When you enter the examination room, you will find a series of 12 booths, known as 'stations'. Each station requires you to undertake a particular task. Some tasks will involve talking to or examining patients, some will involve demonstrating a procedure on an anatomical model.

PLAB Results
During 1996, out of 2982 candidates examined, 1054 (35.3%) passed. Doctors who pass the PLAB test are granted limited registration for 5 years, and are allowed to work in supervised training posts in the UK. Passing the

PLAB is the quickest and least complicated way to obtain GMC registration. In addition, it has the advantage of allowing the doctor to undertake locum work.

Exemption from PLAB

You may apply for exemption from the PLAB (provided you have never attempted it) either:

- through the RCOG's Overseas Doctors Training Scheme (ODTS)

- through the Double Ended Sponsorship Scheme (DESS)

  or

- as a result of sponsorship by some authorized body administering training scheme which has been approved by the GMC, such as the British Council, the Commonwealth Scholarship Commission, the Department of Health, or certain Universities.

The Overseas Doctors Training Scheme (ODTS)

This programme was established by the RCOG in 1984, and is part of the ODTS which is supported by the Department of Health in the UK. It is open to doctors wishing to undergo limited postgraduate training in the British Isles prior to taking the Part 2 examination. During 1997, the RCOG placed 95 overseas doctors in SHO posts in the UK through the ODTS.

Requirements

The requirements for admission to the Sponsorship Scheme are as follows:

1. To have completed 18 months to 2 years post-registration obstetric and gynaecological training in their own country, preferably in RCOG-recognized posts, and have had this training assessed by the Examination Department.

2. To have passed, or been exempted from, the Part 1 examination.

3. To hold a medical qualification registrable with the British GMC or the Irish Registration Council.

5. To have a good standard of written and spoken English. Doctors from non-English speaking countries are usually required to sit the British Council International English Language Testing System (IELTS), medical

module and to score at least 7 in all four components. From January 2000, the IELTS test will be valid for 2 years only. Following that date sponsored doctors whose IELTS test results are more than 2 years old will have to re-sit the test.

6. To be sponsored by the Chairperson of the Representative or Reference Committee in their country. If there is no such committee, then the doctor must be sponsored by a Fellow or Member of the RCOG. In exceptional cases, sponsorship can be from a Dean of a Medical School who is not a Fellow or Member of the College.

Procedure

Candidates wishing to be considered for the Sponsorship scheme and fulfilling the above criteria should write to the Sponsorship Officer at the RCOG, sending their up-to-date curriculum vitae (CV) together with the names and addresses of two referees, preferably Fellows or Members of the College, to whom the Sponsorship Officer will write for confidential reports. Candidates will then be sent the GMC's information sheet and be advised of the names and addresses of the Chairperson of their local RCOG Reference or Representative Committee. Some applicants may prefer to channel their original applications for sponsorship through their local Chairpersons. It is the responsibility of the applicant to request local sponsorship.

The GMC's information sheet must be completed and returned to the College. The College will notify applicants once the GMC provides a decision regarding exemption from the PLAB test. A doctor seeking exemption from the PLAB test must, on arrival to the UK, be capable of performing at least at the level of an experienced SHO in obstetrics and gynaecology and have the ability to perform at the level of a Registrar within 12 months of first taking up an appointment. This exemption is restricted to training in obstetrics and gynaecology only. The GMC will not grant exemption from the PLAB test to doctors who have already taken and failed it. Separate rules regarding medical registration apply in the Republic of Ireland, and the College will advise accordingly if a post is arranged there.

Placement

Once all the requirements are fulfilled the Sponsorship Officer will put the candidate's name on a waiting list to find a suitable training post. The College will send copies of the CV and references to consultants who have expressed a desire to take a sponsored doctor to work in their hospitals. It is essential that the CV is properly typed and correctly set out. An untidy CV will invariably give an impression of careless thinking and disorganized work. Candidates are strongly advised to discuss the content and format of their CVs with their consultants before sending them to the College. As soon as a consultant agrees to appoint a particular trainee, that doctor will be notified by a telegram by the RCOG and will receive an appointment letter from the hospital concerned.

It is the intention of the College to place all sponsored doctors into paid training posts. In certain circumstances, however, if candidates are awarded scholarships from governments or other similar organizations, the RCOG will be in a position to place them into recognized unpaid posts. Most training posts commence on either 1st February or 1st August. The initial appointment could be for either 6 or 12 months duration. Following completion doctors requiring further training must make individual application to advertised posts in open competition.

Duration

Candidates are advised to apply to the College for sponsorship at least 18 months before they hope to start their training in the UK. The average time from completion of formalities to notification of an appointment is variable and depends on the availability of sponsored training posts in the UK. For example, at the beginning of 1999, there were 113 overseas trainees waiting for jobs on the ODTS waiting list. This situation had resulted from the reorganization of the training system in the UK, with the subsequent shortage of salaried posts available for international competition. At that time the College suspended any new additions to the ODTS waiting list till that back log gets cleared. You should contact the ODTS office in the College for the latest situation.

The sponsorship will normally be for a maximum of 2 years, provided that progress is being made and satisfactory reports are received from the consultants with whom the candidate is working.

The Double-Ended Sponsorship Scheme (DESS)

This DESS is a system where named consultants in the UK have established links with, and take on a regular basis from, named consultants or unit overseas known to them personally. Until recently, the candidate seeking exemption from PLAB in this way applied directly to the GMC for limited registration.

When a candidate is personally recommended to the UK consultant, the latter assumes responsibility for the trainee throughout his/her training in the UK. The GMC, however, has recently had cause for concern that in some cases continuing responsibility for the overseas doctor was not being honoured. Consequently, the GMC decided to discontinue this arrangement from April 1994 and directed that the double-ended appointments should be dealt with by the College. As the double-ended scheme has been very successful in the past, the College did not wish to disturb the existing system and, therefore, decided to deal with the DESS applications separately from the ODTS doctors. However, it remains College policy that all doctors applying for posts through the DESS should fulfil the same regulations required of the ODTS doctors.

Beyond the MRCOG

Once the MRCOG is achieved, remember your training has only now started. In the British system, you will not be considered an independent specialist for another 3–4 years at least. There are good reasons for this. Any MRCOG candidate who puts his or her mind to it can theoretically achieve the Part 2 within 2 years of their first SHO job. This does not really give sufficient time for a wide enough experience to fulfil the role of an independent specialist. The post-MRCOG period therefore allows one to gather some general experience and then to subsequently pursue some sub-specialty interest.

Returning home

It is important to plan your return in a constructive way. Too often doctors leave the UK because they had to rather than because they planned to. That is not to say that most overseas doctors wanted to stay in the UK indefinitely, but the timing of their return is forced upon them because their Visa has expired, at a time when they feel they could have done more. It is therefore very important that you realize from the beginning that your time is limited and ensure that you use that time efficiently. This is why planning your stay in the UK is essential. Rest assured that the time allowed is sufficient to achieve a lot as long as it is utilized effectively.

Your return home should be planned from the time you arrived into the UK. This is because you must tailor your experience in the UK to the reality of your home territory. For example, there is scant use for research experience in identifying the HPV type on cervical smears when your community does not even have a cervical screening programme.

What is the niche you are hoping to fill when you return? If you can answer this early, you are in a better position to benefit from your UK experience. Thus, it is essential that you keep in contact with your seniors at home so that they can guide you along. Everyone can presumably do a Caesarean section or a hysterectomy, but what service or expertise can you offer that would make you an asset to your local hospital?

In returning home, you should also try to establish and maintain links with the Department in which you have worked in the UK. This will allow you to continue your relationship and experience even after you have left. When you get home you will realize that the journey has only just begun.

KEY POINTS

- Overseas training in posts assessed and recognized by the College is accepted towards the requirements for the Part 2 examination.

- Some overseas candidates are required to undertake some recognized training in the UK.

- The majority of overseas candidates have to pass, or obtain exemption from, the PLAB test before practising medicine in the UK.

- The Overseas Doctors Sponsorship Scheme and the Double-Ended Sponsorship Scheme provide restricted exemption from the PLAB test and organize recognized training posts for candidates who have passed the Part 1 examination and had had 18–24 months of obstetric and gynaecological training in their own country.

- Overseas candidates requiring information about the PLAB test, medical registration and job opportunities in the UK will find the following addresses useful:

  For initial enquiries
  The First Application Service,
  General Medical Council,
  178 Great Portland Street,
  London W1N 6JE, UK
  Tel: 0171 9153481   Fax: 0171 9153558

For enquiries about job opportunities
National Advice Centre for Postgraduate Medical Education,
The British Council,
Bridgewater House,
58 Whitworth Street,
Manchester Ml 6BB, UK
Tel: 0161 957 7218   Fax: 0161 957 7029

For enquiries about test places and other test details
The PLAB Test Section,
General Medical Council,
178 Great Portland Street,
London WIN 6JE, UK
Te: 0171 915 3727   Fax: 0171 915 3565

For enquiries about IELTS
National Advice Centre for Postgraduate Medical Education,
The British Council,
Bridgewater House,
58 Whitworth Street,
Manchester Ml 6BB, UK
Tel: 0161 957 7755   Fax 0161 957 7762   Email: ed@bdtcoun.org

or

Examinations Services (IELTS),
The British Council,
10 Spring Gardens,
London SW1A 2BN, UK
Tel: 0171 930 8466   Fax: 0171 839 6347

9

Syllabus and Reading

Introduction

Syllabuses and reading lists are usually very contentious issues. As far as the candidates are concerned, a syllabus should have a practical value; it should define clear and achievable standards that candidates can aim for, expect to reach and, having done that, would have a good chance of passing. In this chapter we will first present the syllabus for the Part 2 examination, then explain – in practical terms – how best to achieve the required standards. We will also provide examples of suitable books and journals.

Syllabus for the Part 2 Examination

Candidates are expected to have a comprehensive knowledge of obstetrics and gynaecology and those aspects of medicine, surgery and paediatrics relevant to the practice of both. The Part 2 examination is designed to test the candidates theoretical and practical knowledge of obstetrics and gynaecology. Candidates are expected to show an ability to apply the knowledge of scientific principles previously tested in the Part 1 examination to the management of clinical problems.

Applied Basic Science

Anatomy
Continuing comprehensive knowledge of anatomy, particularly as applied to surgical procedures undertaken by the obstetrician and gynaecologist.

Pathology, biochemistry and endocrinology

Thorough knowledge of the pathology of the genital tract and associated structures; sound understanding of the biochemistry of the mother and fetus, together with in depth knowledge of metabolism. Whilst endocrinological knowledge of all organs is required, extensive knowledge is expected of the endocrine organs as applied to reproductive medicine.

Pharmacology

Comprehensive knowledge of all aspects of pharmacology is required with particular knowledge of those drugs which will be used in obstetrics and gynaecology.

Immunology

Candidates should be expected to understand basic immunology and how this may be changed in pregnancy; fetal development of the immune system, with particular knowledge of rhesus and other iso-immunizations.

Infectious diseases

Comprehensive knowledge of the infectious diseases affecting pregnant and non-pregnant females as well as the fetus in utero. Knowledge of epidemiology, diagnostic techniques, prophylaxis, immunization and the use of antibiotics and antiviral agents.

Epidemiology and statistics

Candidates should understand how to collect data and to apply methods of statistical analysis. They should also have knowledge of setting up clinical trials and the ability to interpret data.

Diagnostic imaging

Understanding of the applications of ultrasound, computerized tomographic scanning and magnetic resonance imaging.

Fetal Medicine

Genetics and embryology

Comprehensive knowledge of normal and abnormal karyotypes, the inheritance of genetic disorders and of the genetic causes of infertility and early abortion. Understanding of the principles of screening for and diagnosis of fetal abnormalities and of the intrauterine treatment of the fetus. Demonstration of the ability to transmit this knowledge to patients and to discuss its practical and ethical implications.

Normal pregnancy

Comprehensive knowledge of maternal and fetal physiology, of antepartum care, its methods of implementation, of intrapartum care, including obstetrical analgesia and anaesthesia, and of the normal puerperium. Understanding of the use of diagnostic testing and of such management strategies as day care and community-based care.

Abnormal pregnancy

Clear knowledge of all aspects of abnormality in pregnancy, labour and puerperium is expected together with their management. Understanding of the effects of pre-existing disease (obstetric, gynaecological or medical) upon pregnancy and demonstration of the ability to provide informative counselling before, during and after pregnancy. Detailed knowledge of neonatal resuscitation and of the principles of neonatal management. Understanding of perinatal pathology.

Maternal and perinatal mortality

Candidates are expected to be familiar with the definitions and concepts as well as to be conversant with confidential enquiries into maternal deaths and the reports on birth surveys.

Pre- and post-pregnancy counselling

Candidates should demonstrate their ability to advise patients regarding any aspect of obstetric or gynaecological disease.

General Gynaecology

Proficiency is expected in taking general and gynaecological histories and in performing general and gynaecological examinations.

Gynaecological surgery

Candidates should understand the uses of day case surgery and of minimally invasive surgery. Detailed knowledge of all basic gynaecological procedures as well as the ability to perform more common gynaecological operations is required, paying particular attention to techniques of incision, closure and drainage of wounds and to the selection of instruments and materials. Candidates will be expected to understand the principles of selection of patients for specific procedures and to have a knowledge of more complicated procedures, e.g. in oncology and infertility, though at the level of the Membership Examination proficiency in these areas will not be expected. Understanding of the complications of surgery and of the principles of postoperative care is also required. There should also be detailed knowledge of the applications, techniques and complications of anaesthesia and of the principles and practice of adult resuscitation, including the use of blood transfusion.

Reproductive Medicine

Prepubertal gynaecology

Thorough knowledge of normal and abnormal sexual development, paediatric pathology and its management, normal puberty and its disorders.

Disorders of menstruation

Based on the physiology of normal menstruation, in-depth understanding of pathophysiology of menstrual disorders, their investigation and management. The menopause and its management.

Infertility

Comprehensive knowledge of the causes of infertility and of the investigations and management of the infertile couple together with basic knowledge of endocrine therapy and of the techniques involved in assisted reproduction.

Contraception and abortion

All methods of contraception should be thoroughly understood and candidates are obliged to present evidence of practical experience. The reasons for, techniques and implications of performing therapeutic abortion should be understood.

Psychosexual medicine

A thorough understanding of the principles of psychosexual medicine is required.

Gynaecological Oncology

Knowledge of the epidemiology and aetiology of gynaecological tumours, of the principles of carcinogenesis, tumour immunology and pathology and of diagnostic techniques and staging of gynaecological tumours is essential. The basic principles of treatment, including surgery, radiotherapy and chemotherapy should be understood together with knowledge of terminal care of patients dying from gynaecological malignancy.

Urogynaecology

Detailed knowledge is required of the presentation and aetiology of urinary symptoms and of catheter management. Understanding of the principles of investigation and of surgical and non-surgical management is expected.

Other Topics

Resource management

Understanding of the provision and rational use of services is expected, together with knowledge of the principles of clinical management and audit.

Ethics and the law

Basic understanding is expected of ethical and legal issues which are involved in contemporary obstetric and gynaecological practice.

Practical scope of the examination

Despite this detailed syllabus, many candidates still find it difficult to practically define the extent of the knowledge required to pass the examination. Phrases such as 'thorough', 'comprehensive', 'in-depth' and 'detailed' are extensively used in the syllabus to describe the required knowledge. However, these phrases are non-specific and tend to suggest that the candidate should know 'everything about everything', which is both unrealistic and untrue. Nevertheless, if we remember two basic facts, it will not be difficult to decide on the exact practical scope of the examination:

1. The examination is aimed at obstetric and gynaecological Specialist Registrars (years 1–3) in the UK and their equivalents. Therefore, *the knowledge expected from you at the examination is similar to what you are expected to know as a Specialist Registrar.* This includes detailed management of the common clinical problems as well as basic management of the less common ones. For example, you will be expected to know the 'ins and outs' of pre-eclampsia, including underlying pathophysiology, symptoms, signs, investigations, antenatal, intrapartum and postpartum management as well as dose, mode of action and side-effects of the drugs used in treatment. On the other hand, no such detailed knowledge will be expected about phaeochromocytoma apart from having a high index of suspicion, initiating the relevant investigations and understanding the basic principles of treatment and the need for referral to a specialist endocrinologist.

2. Your primary aim is to pass the examination, rather than answer *all* the questions (the essay questions are an exception here; you should answer all of them). In fact, very few candidates (and probably Examiners) manage to answer every question. Examiners often deliberately ask questions that have no clear cut answers to see how you will cope in the face of difficulty (a situation not uncommonly encountered in real life). So do not get disheartened if you hear that some Examiners have asked about a rather rare and obscure condition. These questions are almost *never* the cause of failure.

With these two simple facts in mind, we can logically conclude that any postgraduate textbook is suitable for the Part 2 examination, as long as you supplement it with basic understanding of what you do in clinical practice and, more importantly, why you do it.

Suggested reading

Which book to read is mainly a matter of personal choice. The books presented here are for guidance only, and many other books are equally suitable for the preparation for the examination.

You should always read the latest edition of any book. Another important proviso is for candidates reading American books; care is needed because some recommended practices are not those currently used in the UK. The management of some clinical problems may vary considerably across the Atlantic and, as the old saying goes: 'when in Rome do like the Romans do'.

Instead of presenting you with a long formidable list we have divided the books into different categories. Under each category we have explained the role of such books in the preparation for the examination, and provided some examples that have been used previously by successful candidates.

Undergraduate Textbooks

For the uninitiated in obstetrics and gynaecology at the beginning of their training, it is advisable to read first an undergraduate textbook. This will provide an overall view – albeit superficial – of the whole curriculum in a short time and lay down the foundations on which to build more detailed knowledge. It will also give basic definitions (e.g. engagement, presentation, position, vertex). These definitions are common questions in the Part 2 oral assessment examination, but are often assumed and not mentioned in postgraduate textbooks. The textbook you have read as an undergraduate or one of the following examples is suitable.

- Chamberlain GVP (1995) *Ten Teachers.* (Two volumes), London: Edward Arnold.

- Llwellyn-Jones D (1995) *Fundamentals of Obstetrics and Gynaecology*, 6th edition, St. Louis: Mosby.

- Hacker NF and Moore JG (1998) *Essentials of Obstetrics and Gynecology*, 3rd edition, Philadelphia: WB Saunders.

- Symonds EM and Symonds IM (1997) *Essential Obstetrics and Gynaecology*, 3rd edition, Edinburgh: Churchill Livingstone.

- Miller AWF and Hanrethy KP (1997) *Obstetrics Illustrated*, 5th edition, Edinburgh: Churchill Livingstone.

- Govan ADT, McKay Hart D and Callander R (1993) *Gynaecology Illustrated*, 4th edition, Edinburgh: Churchill Livingstone.

Postgraduate Textbooks

These will form the mainstay of your reading for the Membership as well as for your clinical work. Every book has its own style, and you are well advised to read sections from the major textbooks before deciding which one to use. Examples of these books include:

- Whitfield CR (1995) *Dewhurst's Integrated Obstetrics and Gynaecology for Postgraduates*, 5th edition, Oxford: Blackwell Scientific Publications.

- Shaw R, Soutter R and Stanton S (1997) *Gynaecology*, 2nd edition, Edinburgh: Churchill Livingstone.

- Chamberlain GVP (1995) *Turnbull's Obstetrics*, 2nd edition, Edinburgh: Churchill Livingstone.

- Cunningham FG *et al.* (1997) *Williams Obstetrics*, 20th edition, Connecticut: Appleton-Century-Crofts.

- Copeland LJ (1993) *Textbook of Gynecology*, Philadelphia: WB Saunders.

Operative Obstetrics and Gynaecology

Operative obstetrics and gynaecology is part of the syllabus for the examination, but is not usually well-covered by the standard textbooks. The following are examples of suitable operative books.

- Mann WJ and Stovall TG (1996) *Gynaecologic Surgery*, Edinburgh: Churchill Livingstone.

- Thompson JD and Rock JA (1996) *Te Linde's Operative Gynaecology*, 8th edition, Philadelphia: JB Lippincott Company.

- Gershenson DM, De Cherney AH and Curry SL (1993) *Operative Gynaecology*, Philadelphia: WB Saunders.

- Plauché WC, Morrison JC and O'Sullivan MJ (1992) *Surgical Obstetrics*, Philadelphia: WB Saunders.

Anaesthesia and Analgesia

Like all trainees in surgical specialities, you are required to know about the relevant principles and techniques in anaesthesia and analgesia. The following are examples of suitable books.

- Buchan AS and Sharwood-Smith GH (1991) *Handbook of Obstetric Anaesthesia*, London: WB Saunders.

- Dewan DM and Hood DD (1996) *Practical Obstetric Anesthesia*, Philadelphia: WB Saunders.

Multiple Choice Question, OSCE and Case Presentation Books

The knowledge in these books is presented in an examination-like style. They fulfil both educational and self-assessment roles.

- Sharif KW and Jordan JA (1997) *MRCOG Part 2 MCQs - Clinical Obstetrics and Gynaecology*, London: WB Saunders.

- RCOG (1995) *LOGIC MCQ 2nd Series: Obstetrics*, London: RCOG.

- RCOG (1995) *LOGIC MCQ 2nd Series: Gynaecology*, London: RCOG.

- RCOG (1986) *LOGIC MCQ Series: Obstetrics*, London: RCOG.

- RCOG (1987) *LOGIC MCQ Series: Gynaecology*, London: RCOG.

- RCOG (1990) *LOGIC MCQ Series: Reproductive Medicine*, London: RCOG.

- RCOG (1992) *LOGIC MCQ Series: Gynaecological Oncology*, London: RCOG.

- Rymer J and Ahmed H (1998) *OSCEs in Obstetrics and Gynaecology*, Edinburgh: Churchill Livingstone.

- Slade E *et al.* (1994) *Key Questions in Obstetrics and Gynaecology*, London: Bios Scientific Publications.

- Konje JC and Taylor DJ (1998) *OSCE in Obstetrics and Gynaecology,* Oxford: Blackwell Science.

- Baker PN, Fay T and Hammond R (1997) *Obstetrics and Gynaecology - Cases, Questions and Commentaries,* London: WB Saunders.

Other Books
Here are some of the titles that are not 'core' textbooks but, nevertheless, have been found useful by successful candidates.

- Stirrat GM (1997) *Aids to Obstetrics and Gynaecology for MRCOG,* 4th edition, Edinburgh: Churchill Livingstone.

- Nelson-Piercy C (1997) *Handbook of Obstetric Medicine,* Oxford: Isis Medical Media.

- Enkin M *et al.* (1995) *A Guide to Effective Care in Pregnancy and Childbirth,* 2nd edition. Oxford: Oxford University Press.

- Loudon N, Glassier A and Gebbie A (1995) *Handbook of Family Planning and Reproductive Health Care.* 3rd edition, Edinburgh: Churchill Livingstone.

- de Swiet M (1995) *Medical Disorders in Obstetric Practice,* 3rd edition, Oxford: Blackwell Scientific Publications.

- Balen A and Jacobs H (1997) *Infertility in Practice,* Edinburgh: Churchill Livingstone.

- Lumsden MA *et al.* (1997) *Menstrual Problems for the MRCOG,* London: RCOG.

- Dear P and Newell S (1996) *Neonatology for the MRCOG,* London: RCOG.

- Fox H and Buckley H (1998) *Gynaecological and Obstetric Pathology for the MRCOG,* London: RCOG.

- Cardozo L *et al.* (1993) *Basic Urogynaecology,* Oxford: Oxford University Press.

- Kingston H (1997) *ABC of Clinical Genetics,* 2nd edition, London: British Medical Association.

Review Series
Most textbooks are out of date by the time they are published. You are expected to keep abreast of the recent developments in the specialty and should regularly read review series and journals. Examples of review series include the following:

- Studd J. *Progress in Obstetrics and Gynaecology*, Edinburgh: Churchill Livingstone.

- Bonnar J. *Recent Advances in Obstetrics and Gynaecology*, Edinburgh: Churchill Livingstone.

- *Baillière's Clinical Obstetrics and Gynaecology*, London: Baillière Tindall (Various editors).

Journals

Contrary to common belief, it is the general journal *(British Medical Journal, the Lancet)* that is of particular benefit to you in your preparation rather than the specialized one *(British Journal of Obstetrics and Gynaecology, Journal of Obstetrics and Gynaecology, Obstetrics and Gynecology, American Journal of Obstetrics and Gynecology)*. Authors of papers that address important and practical problems are usually interested in these general journals as they have a wider readership. As a result of this, these papers become common knowledge in medicine and you will be expected to know about them. For example, it was the *Lancet* that published the results of the multicentre, multinational study which showed that folic acid reduces the risk of recurrence of neural tube defect (Wald *et al. Lancet* 1991; 338; 131). MRCOG candidates were (and still are) expected to know about these studies. Therefore, you are advised to keep an eye on the *BMJ* and the *Lancet* (available in every postgraduate centre) for at least a year before the examination and read any leading articles or papers with relevance to obstetrics and gynaecology. This is better done prospectively rather than retrospectively 1 month before the examination (an advice often given but rarely followed).

Having done that, you can turn your attention to the specialized journals, particularly the *British Journal of Obstetrics and Gynaecology*. The leading articles and papers should give you an idea on what the College – or at least the Editors of its journal – consider important and topical.

Essential Reading

There is no doubt that the latest *Report on Confidential Enquiries into Maternal Deaths in the United Kingdom* is essential reading for the examination. Every consultant obstetrician and gynaecologist (and Examiner) in the UK gets a free copy, and almost every candidate is asked at least one question about maternal mortality. There is virtually no excuse to do the Part 2 examination not having carefully read this book. It can be easily obtained (or ordered) from any branch of The Stationery Office (website: www.the-stationery-office.co.uk).

KEY POINTS

- The topics covered in the Part 2 MRCOG examination are applied basic science, fetal medicine, general gynaecology, reproductive medicine, gynaecological oncology and urogynaecology.

- The standards of knowledge expected from you at the examination are similar to what a Specialist Registrar in obstetrics and gynaecology working in the UK should know.

- What to read is mainly a personal choice, but your reading should include all the topics covered by the syllabus.

- The latest *Report on Confidential Enquiries into Maternal Deaths in the United Kingdom* is essential reading for the examination.

10

The Examination System

Introduction

Intelligent preparation for the Part 2 examination entails not only acquiring the necessary factual knowledge and clinical experience, but also thorough understanding of the examination format and the marking system. The examination system has recently changed, and it is now almost completely different from what it used to be just a couple of years ago. In this chapter we will provide an overview of the examination format and the marking system.

The examination format

The Part 2 examination has two sections. These will be discussed here in brief to help illustrate the marking system. Full details of both sections are provided in the following chapters.
The two sections are:

1. The written examination: this is held on the Tuesday following the first Monday in March/ September, and consists of three parts:

   - A multiple choice question (MCQ) paper, lasting 2 hours, containing 300 questions in obstetrics and gynaecology.

   - A written paper, lasting 2 hours, of five short answer essay questions primarily concerning obstetrics and those relevant aspects of medicine, surgery, paediatrics and gynaecology.

   - A written paper, lasting 2 hours, of five short answer essay questions primarily concerning gynaecology and those relevant aspects of medicine, surgery and obstetrics.

Full details of the MCQ and essay papers are given in Chapters 11 and 12, respectively.

2. The oral assessment examination: this is held in mid May/November and consists of an assessment circuit containing 12 stations each lasting for 15 minutes. Two stations are 'preparatory', and there is a single Examiner at each of the other 10 stations. Some stations also have a 'role-player'. Full details of the oral assessment examination are given in Chapter 13.

The marking system

The written paper

As described above, the written paper is divided into three parts: one MCQ paper and two short answer essay papers.

The MCQ paper

The MCQ paper is computer-marked out of a total of 100 marks.

The essay papers

There are two essay papers, each containing five questions. Each essay question is marked by a different pair of Examiners out of 10. The mark of each paper is doubled and both are added together to give a total essay mark out of 200. To aid consistency, the Examiners are given written guidelines (from the Examination Committee) on the expected standards of the answers and a structured marking scheme. If the two Examiners cannot agree on a mark, then a third Examiner has a casting vote. Half marks may be used for components within the answer to each question, but the total must be rounded down to a whole mark. For each answer, two marks are allocated for logical coherent expression and overall impression. One or both of these marks may be lost for serious factual errors.

The overall mark of the written paper

The overall mark of the written paper is made of adding up the marks of the MCQ paper and the two essay papers. The MCQ paper contributes one-third (up to 100 marks) and the essay papers contribute two-thirds (up to 200 marks) of the total written paper mark (out of 300 marks). The pass mark is 175. It is not necessary to pass both the MCQ and the essay components, and an overall mark of 175 or more is all that is required. *Only those candidates who achieve this mark or above will proceed to the oral assessment examination.*

The Oral Assessment Examination

Here there are 10 active stations (i.e. with Examiners). Each station is scored out of 10, giving a total mark of 100. The pass mark is 60. For each station, the Examiner is given guidelines on the expected content and standards of the answer, as well as structured marking scheme. This is to aid consistency, but does not mean that Examiners will work to a set script. They have the latitude to explore the candidate's knowledge and understanding.

The results

The results are announced on the Friday of the week of the oral assessment examination. The list of successful candidates is displayed on the notice board in the front hall of the College. From about 18:00 h on the same day (London time) this list is also available on the College website. Individual candidates are notified by first class post (air mail if overseas).

The top candidate (or candidates, if they achieve the same mark) are awarded the gold medal.

Candidates who have taken the examination for the first time and passed with excellent marks are sent a letter of commendation.

Successful candidates are invited to attend the ceremony in the College on the following Friday. Unsuccessful candidates, on the other hand, are sent full details of their marks in the written and oral assessment examination. This is to help them in their preparation for a future examination.

Examinations appeal

Failed candidates wishing to register an appeal on their examination results should notify the College in writing within 21 days of the date of issue of the results. The Chairman of the Examination Committee will review the candidate's performance and, if in his or her opinion, the result is correct the candidate will be informed and advised that a formal appeal may be made to the College.

An appeal panel which will comprise the Chairman of the Examination Committee, one of the College Honorary Officers and an Examiner will be formed and will consider appeals based on the following grounds:

- That there may have been an administrative irregularity or failure in procedure giving rise to reasonable doubt as to the mark obtained, with the effect that the final result would have been different from that issued.

- That there may have been a bias or inadequacy in the assessment of the candidate by one or more of the Examiners.

The Chairman of the Examination Committee will send a copy of the Appeals Procedure to any candidate submitting a request for the result to be re-examined. A fee of £75 will be requested and this will be refunded if the appeal is successful.

KEY POINTS

- The Part 2 MRCOG examination consists of two sections: written and oral assessment examinations. Only those candidates who pass the written examination will proceed to the oral assessment examination.

- The written examination consists of one MCQ paper (100 marks) and two essay papers (200 marks). The pass mark in the written is 175/300.

- The oral assessment examination consists of two preparatory stations and 10 active stations. The pass mark is 60/100.

11

Multiple Choice Questions – Techniques and Examples

Introduction

The written section of the Part 2 examination contains a multiple choice question (MCQ) paper in obstetrics and gynaecology, contributing one-third of the total written examination mark. The paper contains 300 questions and the time allowed is 2 hours.

MCQ format

The MCQs in the Part 2 are in the form of stems, each followed by a *variable* number of branches, and the stem taken together with each branch is counted as a single question. This is different from the usual MCQ style where every stem is always followed by five branches. The branches (rather than the stems, as in the Part 1 examination) are numbered, and there are 300 branches.

The following specimen questions and answers illustrate what you will find in the Part 2 MCQ paper:

Cholestasis of pregnancy is associated with:

1. preterm labour.

2. increased perinatal mortality.

3. increased incidence of postpartum haemorrhage.

Transverse lie of the second twin at term:

4. is an absolute indication for Caesarean section.

Uterine curettage:

5. is associated with an increased incidence of placenta praevia in a subsequent pregnancy.

6. is important in the investigation of secondary infertility.

In the actual examination you will be provided with a computer answer sheet, a special grade HB pencil and a rubber. The answer sheet contains two options for each question: two lozenges labelled **T** (true) and **F** (false). You will be required to indicate whether you knew a particular item to be true or false by blacking out in **bold** either the 'true' or 'false' lozenge. *The whole lozenge should be blacked out.* Other marks like **X** or √ are not recognized by the computer.

You must use only the grade HB pencil provided for completing all parts of the answer sheets. This is essential as the answer sheets are marked by a computer that is programmed to recognize the shade of this pencil mark.

A few weeks before the examination date you will receive (with your entry card) detailed instructions from the RCOG on how to complete the your answer sheet. You are strongly advised to read these instructions thoroughly and acquaint yourself with their details. The examination hall is not the ideal place to be reading answering instructions for the first time. Detailed instructions and sample answer sheet for the MCQ papers in the Part 2 examination are provided in Appendix 3.

The marking system

The answer sheets are marked by computer. Each item correctly answered (whether it is 'true' or 'false') is awarded one mark (+1). For each incorrect answer no marks are awarded or deducted (0).

MCQ techniques

These have been described in detail in Chapter 4, which you are advised to read again when preparing for the MCQ in the Part 2 examination. A reminder of the important and relevant points is given here.

Read Carefully and Understand Clearly

Read the question carefully and make sure you understand it. Do not simply *think* you understand it. In the Part 2 MRCOG, when you have to go through 300 items in 2 hours, it is not uncommon to rush in and misread the questions. 'Pre-eclampsia' could be easily misread as 'eclampsia', 'morbidity' as 'mortality' and 'fetal haemoglobin' as 'fetal blood'. The opening stem should be read together with each of the branches and taken as a single item. Each item should be considered independently of the other statements.

Do Not Read Between the Lines

Accept the question at face value and do not look for catches or hidden meanings. Trust that the Examiners are trying to test your factual knowledge, not to trick you into making mistakes. What you clearly understand from the question is what is meant by it.

To Guess or Not To Guess

After reading (and understanding) each item, your initial response will fall into one of three categories.

Firstly – you may be sure of the answer and have no doubt about the correct response (whether true or false) – go ahead and without hesitation answer the question.

Secondly, there are those items about which you are not quite certain and yet they 'ring a bell'. You may not immediately know the answer, but from your basic knowledge you could reason it out from first principles – go for it and play your hunches. Such educated hunches that are based on sound judgment and reasoning are more often right than wrong, and you are advised to be bold and answer these items accordingly.

Thirdly, you may be totally ignorant of the answer. The usual advice in such situations, with the *negative* marking system used in many MCQ examinations, is not to guess. However, in the Part 2 MRCOG examination this system has been abolished since 1994. There is nothing to be lost by blindly guessing the answers to such items. If you are incorrect you will not lose any marks and if you are correct (50% probability) you will gain. Readers who are preparing for other examinations which still use the negative marking system should not guess blindly.

Organize Your Time

In the Part 2 MRCOG examination you are allowed 2 hours for 300 questions. This might appear too little, but it is not. The items you are sure of will take only a few seconds. The same applies to those items about which you are totally ignorant. We suggest you go through the whole paper first, answering those questions to which you are sure you know the answers. As you are unlikely to change these answers, you are advised to record them on the answer sheet from the outset. The remaining time should be directed to the unanswered, more time-consuming items about which you are uncertain but have enough basic knowledge to make reasoned hunches. You should have marked these items on the question paper during your first reading to facilitate coming back to them. Any remaining time should be spent on revising the answers, but remember that your first thought is likely to be the correct answer.

Fill-in the Answer Sheet Correctly

A sure recipe for disaster in MCQ examinations is to make a systematic error in recording the answers. If you answer question 1 in place of question 2, all the following answers will also be recorded wrongly. Such mistakes are quite easily done under the stress of the examination. Make sure when you fill-in every answer that it is in the right place.

MCQ Terminology

This has been described in Chapter 4.

Practising MCQs

This is as important as reading textbooks. Some MCQ books are listed in Chapter 10. Other examination-styled MCQ are provided at the end of this chapter. You should use these for self-assessment, i.e. attempt to answer the questions before looking at the provided answers.

KEY POINTS

- The MCQ papers form one-third of the written section of the Part 2 examination.

- When answering an MCQ, read the stem and each option carefully, understand them clearly and consider them independently of other options.

- Take each question at its face value.

- Work out the answers by educated reasoning from basic principles.

- If you do not know the answer, guess. There is no negative marking system in the Part 1 examination. If you guess an answer there is (at least theoretically) a 50% chance of getting it right, and nothing to lose.

- Aim to score as high as possible and do not assume that there is a safe score above which you do not need to attempt any more questions.

- Mark your answers clearly and accurately and keep an eye on the time.

Example MCQ Examinations

The following practice MCQ are similar to the Part 2 questions in content and format. However, although in the actual examination there is a variable number of branches after each stem, we have elected here to have five branches after each stem. This allows more questions to be asked about each subject, and hence more practice. These questions are arranged in four 150-MCQ papers; two in obstetrics and two in gynaecology. An obstetrics paper and a gynaecology paper could be regarded as an examination. The answers are provided at the end of this chapter, but before looking them up you are advised to try to answer the questions from your knowledge. Try to practice against the clock, giving 1 hour for each paper.

Paper 1–Obstetrics:
With regard to oblique lie of the fetus:

1. the incidence is unaffected by parity.

2. at term dorso-anterior are more frequent than dorso-posterior positions.

3. in labour there is a recognized indication for classical Caesarean section.

4. there is a recognized association with fetal renal agenesis.

5. prolapse of an arm occurs more frequently than prolapsed cord.

There is a recognized association between Down's syndrome and:

6. atrial septal defect.

7. congenital deafness.

8. a chromosomal translocation defect.

9. a single palmar crease.

10. clinodactyly of the 5th finger.

Chorioamnionitis:

11. is a recognized cause of preterm labour.

12. does not occur in the absence of maternal pyrexia.

13. is associated with the use of fetal scalp electrode.

14. can usually be prevented by the use of prophylactic penicillin.

15. occurring before the 24th week of pregnancy, fetal sepsis accounts for 75% of perinatal morbidity and mortality.

Drugs considered to be unsuitable for administration to the breast-feeding mother include:

16. nalidixic acid.

17. clonidine hydrochloride.

18. rifampicin.

19. senna.

20. lithium carbonate.

Recognized causes of vomiting in the second trimester of pregnancy include:

21. ectopic gestation.

22. herpes gestationis.

23. ulcerative colitis.

24. acute pyelonephritis.

25. necrobiosis in a fibromyoma.

Dystocia is a characteristic feature of labour in a woman with:

26. a mento-posterior position.

27. a breech presentation.

28. an android pelvis.

29. electrolyte imbalance.

30. cervical fibroid.

The mean birth weight at term is:

31. increased in Beckwith-Wiedemann syndrome.

32. depressed by cigarette smoking in pregnancy.

33. decreased with parity.

34. usually reduced in uncontrolled diabetes mellitus.

35. higher in male as compared with female infants.

Recognized complications of external cephalic version include:

36. a positive Kleihauer–Betke test.

37. fetal bradycardia.

38. uterine rupture.

39. cord presentation.

40. fetal death.

Neonatal jaundice appearing on the third day and still present at 2 weeks of age may be due to:

41. haemolytic disease of the newborn due to rhesus incompatibility.

42. galactosaemia.

43. atresia of the bile duct.

44. phenylketonuria.

45. neonatal hyperthyroidism.

In the pregnant woman aged 35 years or over there is an increased incidence of:

46. macrosomia.

47. intrauterine growth retardation.

48. postmaturity.

49. breech presentation.

50. chromosomal abnormalities.

Oligohydramnios is characteristically associated with:

51. diabetes mellitus.

52. rhesus iso-immunization.

53. fetal renal agenesis.

54. haemangioma of the placenta.

55. fetal duodenal atresia.

In relation to drug treatment during pregnancy:

56. chlorpropamide may cause neonatal hypoglycaemia.

57. propranolol does not affect the fetal heart rate.

58. chlorothiazide can cause maternal pancreatitis.

59. warfarin is a recognized cause of fetal abnormality.

60. thyroxine is likely to cause neonatal hyperthyroidism.

Abnormally high concentration of human chorionic gonadotrophin (HCG) in pregnancy is associated with:

61. multiple pregnancy.

62. fetal erythroblastosis.

63. carneous mole.

64. iniencephaly.

65. Down's syndrome.

Forty patients participated in a randomized controlled trial of complete bed rest versus ambulation in the management of proteinuric hypertension during pregnancy. The measurements of urinary oestriol (nmol/l) in the two groups were as follows:

	Rested Group ($n = 20$)	Ambulant Group ($n = 20$)
Mean	209.9	365.6
S.D.	270.3	197.1
Range	1020	745
$t = 2.08$	Difference between means = 155.7	$P = 0.022$

The following statements, which refer to the above data, are true:

66. the standard error of the mean for the rested group was 270.3.

67. the value of the '*t*' refers to a test for the difference between the means.

68. the value $P = 0.022$ suggests that the observed differences did not occur by chance.

69. in the ambulant group, 95% of the oestriol values were between 365.6 ± 197.1.

70. in the study described, patients were allocated alternately to 'ambulant' and 'rested' groups.

The following are typically inherited as an X–linked trait:

71. achondoplasia.

72. Huntington chorea.

73. glucose-6-phosphate dehydrogenase deficiency.

74. von Willebrand's disease.

75. haemophilia A.

In pregnancy complicated by insulin-dependent maternal diabetes mellitus:

76. the risk of intrauterine death of the fetus is greatest during the last 4 weeks of pregnancy.

77. the insulin requirement may decrease during the first trimester.

78. an increase in the incidence of fetal abnormality is found with mild hypoglycaemia.

79. oral hypoglycaemic agents do not cross the placenta.

80. there is increased incidence of dystocia.

In the amniotic fluid:

81. lecithin contributes nearly 70% of surfactants at 38 weeks' gestation.

82. phospholipids make up more than 80% of surfactants.

83. the bilirubin concentration is higher in the second trimester as compared with the third trimester.

84. phosphotidylinositol is present only if the fetus is mature.

85. a lecithin:sphingomyelin ratio of 2:1 indicates fetal lung maturity in maternal diabetes.

Cholestasis of pregnancy:

86. characteristically appears in the third trimester.

87. has a racial variation.

88. is characteristically associated with neonatal jaundice.

89. pruritis in the absence of jaundice is the most common symptom.

90. is associated with premature labour.

Maternal urinary oestriol excretion during the last trimester of pregnancy is lowered:

91. in multiple pregnancy.

92. by ampicillin therapy

93. during mandelamine therapy.

94. with bed rest.

95. in patients with placental sulphatase deficiency.

In a 38-year-old woman, who continues with the pregnancy after unsuccessful postcoital contraception:

96. the risk of Down's Syndrome is less than 1%.

97. the risk of fetal abnormalities is 20%.

98. cordocentesis is safer than amniocentesis.

99. there is a 10-fold increase in the risk of neural tube defect as compared with a woman aged 25.

100. termination of pregnancy should be advised.

Dizygotic twins:

101. have an increased incidence with maternal age.

102. in labour, the first twin is most commonly in breech presentation.

103. have an incidence which varies with ethnic group.

104. have a higher perinatal mortality if they are of different sex.

105. intrauterine growth retardation is a recognized feature.

Anaemia in pregnancy:

106. MCV (mean corpuscular volume) is the most sensitive indicator of iron deficiency anaemia.

107. serum ferritin is increased in iron deficiency anaemia.

108. red cell folate level is a more sensitive indicator of folate deficiency as compared with serum folate levels.

109. a normal MCV excludes folate deficiency.

110. parenteral administration of iron leads to haemosidrosis in the infant.

The following are recognized causes of postpartum collapse in the absence of significant external bleeding:

111. intravenous ergometrine.

112. eclampsia.

113. uterine rupture.

114. uterine inversion.

115. ischiorectal haematoma.

There is an increased incidence of prolapse of the umbilical cord with:

116. increasing maternal age.

117. postmaturity.

118. high parity.

119. breech presentation.

120. Kielland forceps delivery.

Congenital uterine abnormalities in pregnancy are associated with an increased incidence of:

121. habitual abortion.

122. premature labour.

123. breech presentation.

124. pre-eclampsia.

125. polyhydramnios.

There is an increased incidence of the following conditions during the puerperium as compared with pregnancy:

126. thyroiditis.

127. perforated peptic ulcer.

128. torsion of an ovarian cyst.

129. thromboembolism.

130. psychosis.

Early decelerations of the fetal heart rate in labour:

131. reach their lowest amplitude with the peak of uterine contractions.

132. indicate fetal hypokalaemia.

133. are a sign of fetal hypoxia.

134. indicate fetal distress if they occur repeatedly.

135. are due to cord compression.

Characteristic features of megaloblastic anaemia in pregnancy include:

136. raised serum vitamin B_{12} concentration.

137. reduced red cell folate concentration.

138. glossitis.

139. increased clearance of intravenously injected folic acid.

140. increased lobulation on the nuclei of neutrophils.

A 24-year-old primigravida at 37 weeks gestation had a blood pressure of 150/100 mmHg and 4 g of proteinuria for the preceding 7 days. The following findings would be expected:

141. raised plasma urate levels.

142. loss of diurnal variation in blood pressure.

143. a creatinine clearance of 120–150 ml/min.

144. hyperreflexia.

145. a lowered level of fibrinogen degradation products.

There is a recognized association between Down's syndrome and:

146. trisomy 13.

147. congenital duodenal atresia.

148. hypotonia.

149. leukaemia.

150. advanced paternal age.

Paper 2–Obstetrics:

Features of disseminated intravascular coagulation include:

151. thrombocytopaenia.

152. impairment of myometrial function.

153. reversal of the process by transfusion of stored whole blood.

154. raised fibrinogen levels.

155. always a secondary phenomenon.

Serum alpha-feto protein (AFP) concentration is raised:

156. in the presence of congenital adrenal hyperplasia.

157. in women taking oral contraceptives.

158. in the presence of closed spina bifida.

159. in the presence of fetal exomphalos.

160. after amniocentesis.

An increased intake of folic acid is required when pregnancy is associated with:

161. the administration of anticonvulsants.

162. the administration of ampicillin.

163. sickle cell disease.

164. multiple gestation.

165. the use of co-trimoxazole.

In patients with gestational diabetes:

166. there is a history of parental diabetes mellitus in approximately 50% of cases.

167. serial estimations of maternal glycosylated haemoglobin (HbA1c) concentration are of value in assessing biochemical control.

168. the appearance of ketonuria in the presence of normal blood glucose concentrations indicates the need for an increase in dietary carbohydrate.

169. continuation of pregnancy beyond 38 weeks is contraindicated.

170. impaired glucose tolerance persists after delivery in the majority of women.

The following conditions can be diagnosed directly by ultrasonic visualization of the fetus:

171. congenital heart block.

172. hydrops fetalis.

173. epidermolysisi bullosa dystrophica.

174. Down's syndrome.

175. duodenal atresia.

Perinatal mortality:

176. is defined as the number of stillbirths plus neonatal deaths in the first 28 days of life.

177. is higher in lower socioeconomic classes.

178. is increased in heavy smokers.

179. is lower in nulliparous women compared with those having their second child.

180. is higher in multiple pregnancy.

Suppression of lactation with bromocriptine:

181. is a recognized cause of hypotension.

182. should be given for 1 week only.

183. the effect of the above treatment can be augmented by the concomitant administration of metoclopramide.

184. is not indicated in a women with a stillborn baby under 28 weeks gestation.

185. predisposes to deep venous thrombosis.

Listeria monocytogenes:

186. is a Gram-positive coccus.

187. grows in cold environment.

188. is found in the soil.

189. when acquired transplacentally, neonatal respiratory problems are present in over 90% of cases.

190. is susceptible to ampicillin.

There is a recognized association between intrauterine death of the fetus and:

191. cytomegalovirus infection.

192. sickle cell trait.

193. maternal infection with poliomyelitis.

194. maternal diabetes mellitus.

195. external cephalic version.

True proteinuria in pregnancy is a characteristic feature of:

196. chronic glomerulonephritis.

197. essential benign hypertension.

198. acute pyelonephritis.

199. placental abruption without pre-eclampsia.

200. systemic lupus erythematosus.

The following conditions are associated with an increased incidence of preterm labour:

201. previous cryosurgery to the cervix.

202. fetal oesophageal atresia.

203. prelabour rupture of the membranes.

204. asymptomatic bacteriuria.

205. the presence of fetal fibronectin in cervical and vaginal secretions during the first trimester.

The following statements regarding the maternal cardiovascular system in pregnancy are correct:

206. supraventricular arrhythmias occur with greater frequency than in the non-pregnant woman.

207. the systemic vascular resistance is reduced by 30% in the second trimester.

208. most murmurs detected for the first time during pregnancy are due to increased blood flow across the pulmonary valve.

209. in patients with chronic mitral valve disease crystalline penicillin provides adequate antibiotic prophylaxis at the time of delivery.

210. frusemide is contraindicated for the treatment of heart failure.

With regard to Down's syndrome due to translocation – t(21;21):

211. there is an increased incidence with advanced maternal age.

212. if one parent is a carrier of the balanced translocation, the risk of an affected fetus is at least 1 in 2.

213. it accounts for 95% of all cases of Down's syndrome.

214. the overall incidence is 1 in 800 liveborn infants.

215. there is an increased incidence of Hirschsprung's disease.

Regarding maternal thyrotoxicosis complicating pregnancy and the puerperium:

216. drug therapy can be reliably monitored by serial estimation of total serum thyroxine concentration alone.

217. anti-thyroid drugs should be replaced by propranolol in the last 4 weeks of pregnancy.

218. neonatal goitre is a recognised complication of overtreatment with anti-thyroid drugs.

219. breast feeding is contraindicated if the mother is taking propylthiouracil.

220. when mild, it is difficult to distinguish from the normal physiological changes in the mid trimester.

Sickle cell disease in pregnancy is associated with:

221. increased maternal mortality.

222. neonatal sickle cell crisis.

223. fat embolism.

224. pre-eclampsia.

225. haematuria.

Toxoplasmosis in pregnancy:

226. the incidence of congenital toxoplasmosis in the UK is 2 per 1000 births.

227. is treated with spiramycin.

228. chorioretinitis is the most common neonatal manifestation.

229. acute infection can be diagnosed by the presence of specific IgM antibodies in maternal blood.

230. is transmitted by cats.

Cytomegalovirus infection:

231. is the commonest congenital infection in the UK.

232. can be diagnosed in the neonate by culture of urine.

233. is associated with intracerebral calcification.

234. causes microcephaly.

235. is rare if the mother is immune prior to pregnancy.

In breast-feeding mothers, the following drugs are not contraindicated:

236. warfarin.

237. tetracycline.

238. pethidine.

239. tricyclic antidepressants.

240. reserpine.

Rupture of the uterus is associated with:

241. fetal distress.

242. haematuria.

243. slow pulse rate.

244. intraperitoneal haemorrhage.

245. hypotension.

Ambiguous genitalia at birth are associated with:

246. congenital adrenal hyperplasia.

247. Klinefelter's syndrome.

248. maternal polycystic ovarian disease.

249. maternal administration of sex steroids.

250. Turner's syndrome.

Administration of a bolus dose of oxytocin in the third stage of labour is associated with:

251. increased cardiac output.

252. reduced peripheral resistance.

253. nausea and vomiting.

254. increased central venous pressure.

255. reduced vaginal blood loss.

There is a recognized association between pulmonary embolism and:

256. advanced maternal age.

257. multiparity.

258. severe iron deficiency anaemia.

259. preterm labour.

260. blood group O.

Reduced uteroplacental blood flow can be caused by:

261. intermittent positive pressure ventilation.

262. epidural anaesthesia.

263. aortic compression syndrome.

264. anterior placenta.

265. the use of aspirin.

Epidural anaesthesia is contraindicated in:

266. pre-eclampsia.

267. breech presentation.

268. patients on anticoagulant therapy.

269. local sepsis.

270. preterm labour.

Massive pulmonary embolism with central involvement is associated with:

271. sinus tachycardia.

272. signs of right-sided heart strain.

273. chest X-ray with signs of pulmonary congestion.

274. cyanosis.

275. ischaemic cardiac pain.

Congenital dislocation of the hip is associated with:

276. female infant.

277. family history.

278. polyhydramnios.

279. breech presentation.

280. induction of ovulation.

An increased incidence of postpartum haemorrhage is found in:

281. multiparity.

282. instrumental delivery.

283. the use of an oxytocic drug for the third stage of labour.

284. haemophilia A carriers.

285. Marfan's syndrome.

The following are recognized indications for classical Caesarean section:

286. postmortem operation.

287. previous classical operation.

288. transverse lie.

289. Caesarean section with tubal ligation.

290. Caesarean hysterectomy for cervical cancer.

The following conditions are transmitted as autosomal recessive:

291. Ehler–Danlos syndrome.

292. spherocytosis.

293. Tay–Sachs disease.

294. cystic fibrosis.

295. tuberous sclerosis.

The incidence of respiratory distress syndrome:

296. may be reduced by antenatal administration of steroids.

297. is higher in female infants.

298. is increased in term babies whose weight is below the 10th centile.

299. is lower in babies delivered by elective Caesarean section.

300. is lower in babies born to heroin-addicted mothers.

Paper 3–Gynaecology:

Barr body is found in:

301. Klinefelter's syndrome.

302. Turner's syndrome.

303. male Down's syndrome.

304. adrenogenital syndrome.

305. pituitary hypoplasia.

Regarding pituitary prolactinoma:

306. bromocriptine is contraindicated.

307. causes binasal hemianopia.

308. causes impotence in the male.

309. prolactin level is depressed in pregnancy.

310. may increase in size in pregnancy.

Regarding hydatidiform mole:

311. the incidence increases over the age of 40.

312. the karyotype is usually 46XY.

313. it causes unilateral ovarian cysts.

314. in the complete mole variety, there is raised serum AFP.

315. it is more common in patient–consort pairs of blood groups A-O.

Adrenal tumours with hirsutism are associated with:

316. loss of the circadian rhythm.

317. increased plasma levels of adrenocorticotropic hormone (ACTH).

318. hyperglycaemia.

319. increased plasma levels of 17-hydroxyprogesterone.

320. increased urinary levels of 17-ketosteroids.

Painless haematuria occurs in:

321. acute urinary tract infection.

322. interstitial cystitis.

323. carcinoma of the bladder.

324. incompatible blood transfusion.

325. rifampicin therapy.

Granulosa cell tumours:

326. occur in all age groups.

327. are commonly bilateral.

328. are malignant in 30% of cases.

329. are associated with Call–Exner bodies.

330. are associated with carcinoma of the endometrium.

In polycystic ovarian disease:

331. serum follicle-stimulating hormone (FSH) is raised.

332. serum sex hormone-binding globulin (SHBG) is raised.

333. there are multiple corpus luteal cysts in the ovary.

334. serum androstenedione is raised.

335. there is associated hyperinsulinaemia.

The following are correct associations:

336. Klinefelter's syndrome – normal testosterone levels.

337. Turner's syndrome – 46XO.

338. true gonadal dysgenesis – 46XY.

339. female adrenogenital syndrome – 46XX.

340. triple X syndrome (superfemale) – 46XXX.

Oligospermia is characteristically associated with:

341. bronchiectasis.

342. cryptochidism.

343. sulphasalazine therapy.

344. heavy smoking.

345. alcohol consumption.

Recognized side effects of the administration of danazol include:

346. dizziness.

347. dryness of the vagina.

348. decrease in breast size.

349. acne.

350. hirsutism.

With regard to dystrophies of the vulva:

351. malignant changes occur in more than 10% of cases of 'leukoplakia'.

352. there is familial predisposition to lichen sclerosus.

353. topical testosterone is a recognized treatment for lichen sclerosus.

354. pruritis is a recognized feature of carcinoma in situ.

355. the clitoris is rarely involved in hypertrophic dystrophy.

Anorexia nervosa is characterized by:

356. a low basal serum luteinizing hormone (LH) concentration.

357. loss of body hair.

358. loss of appetite.

359. prompt return of menstruation as soon as body weight approaches normal level.

360. suicide as a common cause of death.

Recognized side-effects of clomiphene citrate include:

361. ascites.

362. loss of head hair.

363. hypotension.

364. hot flushes.

365. blurring of vision.

Premature ovarian failure:

366. is a recognized complication of mumps.

367. is a characteristic feature of anorexia nervosa.

368. may run an intermittent course.

369. is associated with autoimmune disease.

370. is associated with elevated levels of serum calcium.

Pain originating in a uterine fibroid is associated with:

371. sarcomatous changes.

372. infection.

373. endometrial carcinoma.

374. red degeneration.

375. torsion of a pedunculated fibroid.

In a 25-year-old woman, serum FSH concentration is raised in:

376. polycystic ovarian disease.

377. cystadinocarcinoma of the ovary.

378. ovarian agenesis.

379. long-term administration of luteinizing hormone-releasing hormone (LHRH) analogues.

380. hydatidiform mole.

The following are recognized features of septic abortion:

381. hypotension.

382. acute renal failure.

383. disseminated intravascular coagulation.

384. jaundice.

385. crepitus.

Increased incidence of endometrial carcinoma is associated with:

386. prolonged use of the combined oral contraceptive pill.

387. polycystic ovarian disease.

388. late menopause.

389. obesity.

390. multiparity.

The following are correct associations:

391. stage Ic ovarian carcinoma – ascites.

392. stage III endometrial carcinoma – involvement of bladder mucosa.

393. stage III vulval carcinoma – bilateral regional lymph node metastasis.

394. stage IIa cervical carcinoma – involvement of the lower third of the vagina.

395. stage III vaginal carcinoma – extension on to the pelvic wall.

Procedures of value in the diagnosis of gonorrhoea in the female include:

396. culture of high vaginal swab.

397. naked-eye examination of the vaginal discharge.

398. examination of the male partner.

399. gonococcal complement fixation test.

400. culture of urethral swab.

The aims of surgery for the relief of female stress incontinence of urine include:

401. elevation of the bladder neck above the pelvic diaphragm.

402. correction of funnelling at the bladder neck.

403. increasing urethral resistance.

404. increasing detrusor stability.

405. reduction of the functional length of the urethra.

Recognized causes of galactorrhoea include:

406. dysgerminoma of the ovary.

407. acromegaly.

408. methyl-dopa.

409. hyperthyroidism.

410. chronic renal failure.

The following syndromes or lesions are correctly paired with a recognized association:

411. choriocarcinoma – hyperthyroidism.

412. anorexia nervosa – loss of head hair.

413. acute retention of urine – haemorrhoidectomy.

414. treatment of anovulation – ascites.

415. hypertension – administration of bromocriptine.

Recognized side-effects of cyclophosphamide include:

416. neuropathy.

417. alopecia.

418. haemorrhagic cystitis.

419. pulmonary fibrosis.

420. hypermagnesaemia.

The following are recognized associations:

421. fibroids – polycythaemia.

422. hyperprolactinaemia – increased incidence of breast cancer.

423. vasectomy – antisperm antibodies.

424. Sertoli-cell-only syndrome – elevated FSH and LH.

425. endometriosis – infertility.

Presumptive evidence of ovulation include:

426. biphasic temperature chart.

427. subnuclear vaculation in endometrial cells.

428. raised progesterone levels in the second half of the menstrual cycle.

429. ferning of cervical mucus.

430. positive spinnbarkeit test.

Chlamydial infection:

431. is caused by a Gram-positive intracellular organism.

432. is sensitive to cephalosporins.

433. is usually asymptomatic.

434. causes lymphogranuloma inguinale.

435. is a recognized cause of perihepatitis.

Female genital tuberculosis:

436. is usually a primary infection of the Fallopian tubes.

437. the ovaries are involved in 30% of cases.

438. is a recognized cause of ascites.

439. is associated with infertility due to tubal blockage.

440. causes infertility which is reversible with modern chemotherapy.

With regard to the climacteric:

441. the mean age of the menopause in the UK is 48 years.

442. there is a decrease in prolactin levels.

443. there is a high risk of malignant changes in fibroids.

444. there is a decrease in serum calcium levels.

445. there are high levels of gonadotrophins which are maintained indefinitely.

The following are associated with early menopause:

446. early menarche.

447. multiparity.

448. cigarette smoking.

449. obesity.

450. familial deletion of qX.

Paper 4–Gynaecology:

The following hormones are active when given orally:

451. progesterone.

452. oestradiol benzoate.

453. ethinyl oestradiol.

454. norethisterone.

455. conjugated equine oestrogen.

Therapeutic indications for progestogens include:

456. endometriosis.

457. fibroids.

458. endometrial carcinoma.

459. habitual abortion.

460. dysfunctional uterine bleeding.

The following are recognized causes for delay in the recovery of consciousness after general anaesthesia:

461. fat embolism.

462. acute intermittent porphyria.

463. phaeochromocytoma.

364. residual curarisation.

465. anoxia during anaesthesia.

Ovarian theca cell tumours:

466. are a recognized cause of Meigs' syndrome.

467. are usually benign.

468. are found in postmenopausal women.

469. are typically found in prepubertal girls.

470. are bilateral in over 20% of cases.

As compared with radiotherapy, radical hysterectomy for cervical carcinoma:

471. causes more dysapreunia.

472. is more likely to cause damage to the ureters.

473. is preferred for young patients with stage Ib disease.

474. has a higher treatment-associated mortality.

475. causes lymphocysts more frequently.

With radiotherapy for the treatment of cervical carcinoma:

476. survival of normal cells is improved with treatment with hyperbaric oxygen.

477. the bowel mucosa is more sensitive than the bladder mucosa.

478. it is the treatment of choice for stage III disease.

479. the risk of complications is reduced if the radiotherapy is combined with surgery.

480. pulmonary embolism is a recognized complication.

Triple X syndrome:

481. has an incidence of 1 in 10 000 female births.

482. its incidence increases with maternal age.

483. is associated with low intelligence.

484. has characteristic phenotypical abnormalities.

485. results from non-disjunction.

Progesterone-only pill:

486. inhibits ovulation in more than 60% of users.

487. leads to menstrual irregularities.

488. reduces the incidence of functional ovarian cysts.

489. is contraindicated in smokers over the age of 35.

490. when discontinued, the return of fertility is more rapid as compared with the combined oral contraceptive pill.

Vasectomy:

491. is the contraceptive method used by 15% of couples worldwide.

492. may be performed under local anaesthesia.

493. has a failure rate of 2–4 per 1000 procedures.

494. is effective within 2 weeks of the procedure.

495. is associated with the production of antisperm antibodies in over 50% of men.

The following drugs may cause male subfertility:

496. cimetidine.

497. sulphasalazine.

498. imipramine.

499. thiazide diuretics.

500. spironolactone.

The following may be associated with Meigs' syndrome:

501. cystadenoma.

502. thecoma.

503. granulosa cell tumour.

504. Brenner's tumour.

505. fibroma.

Fallot's tetralogy is associated with:

506. central cyanosis.

507. atrial septal defect.

508. aortic stenosis.

509. right ventricular hypertrophy.

510. ejection systolic murmur.

Wound dehiscence

511. occurs more frequently in a Pfannenstiel incision as compared with a vertical midline incision.

512. is reduced with mass closure technique.

513. is increased with early postoperative mobilization.

514. is increased in obese patients.

515. usually occurs between the 5th and 10th postoperative days.

Raised serum AFP is associated with:

516. hepatocellular carcinoma.

517. leiomyosarcoma.

518. endodermal sinus tumour.

519. immature teratoma.

520. viral hepatitis.

With regard to female laparoscopic sterilization:

521. reversal is successful in 95% of cases.

522. clips should be applied to the infundibular part of the tube.

523. should not be performed when the patient is having a period.

524. the failure rate with Filshie clips is 1–2 per 1000.

525. the associated mortality rate is 8–10 per 1000 procedures.

Recognized side-effects of cisplatin include:

526. hypercalcaemia.

527. papillitis.

528. ototoxicity.

529. myelosuppression.

530. hypomagnesaemia.

Recognized causes of cystic swellings within the female breast include:

531. hyperprolactinaemia.

532. degeneration within a colloid carcinoma.

533. fibroadenosis.

534. chronic abscess.

535. galactocele.

The following are correct associations:

536. androgen insensitivity – hirsutism.

537. single gonadotrophin deficiency – anosmia.

538. polycystic ovarian disease – dysfunctional uterine bleeding.

539. Klinefelter's syndrome – 47XXY.

540. Turner's syndrome – lymphoedema.

Diethylstilboestrol (DES) exposure during pregnancy may lead to:

541. oligospermia in male offspring.

542. vaginal adenosis in female offspring.

543. increased spontaneous abortion in female offspring.

544. increased risk of breast cancer.

545. urogenital structural abnormalities in female offspring.

Mifepristone (RU486):

546. blocks the action of progesterone at the receptor level.

547. when administered in the first 3 days of the follicular phase, leads to inhibition of ovulation in 50% of users.

548. in combination with prostaglandins, it causes complete abortion in 95% of women with early pregnancy.

549. crosses the placenta.

550. its use for termination of pregnancy is contraindicated if fetal heart action is detected by ultrasound.

A woman who conceived with an intrauterine contraceptive device in situ has an increased risk of:

551. congenitally malformed fetus.

552. ectopic pregnancy.

553. preterm labour.

554. complications of the third stage of labour.

555. hydatidiform mole.

The following are correct associations:

556. stage IV ovarian carcinoma – superficial liver metastases.

557. stage IIIa endometrial carcinoma – para-aortic lymph nodes metastases.

558. stage IVa vulval carcinoma – invasion of the upper urethra.

559. stage IIb cervical carcinoma – parametrial involvement.

560. stage II vaginal carcinoma – involvement of the subvaginal tissue.

The following patients with genital prolapse should preferably be treated conservatively:

561. patients who are within 3 months after childbirth.

562. patients with a prolapse after total abdominal hysterectomy.

563. patients with complete procidentia.

564. patients with enterocoele.

565. patients with severe respiratory compromise.

Recognized features of Turner's syndrome include:

566. coarctation of the aorta.

567. anosmia.

568. increased incidence with advanced maternal age.

569. hypogonadotrophic hypogonadism.

570. increased carrying angle.

With regard to transection of the ureter discovered during abdominal hysterectomy:

571. end-to-end anastomosis is contraindicated.

572. if the other kidney is present, the damaged ureter should be ligated.

573. repair should be performed using absorbable sutures.

574. the Boari flap procedure is a recognized method of treatment.

575. the site of injury should be drained and the repair delayed for 2 weeks.

Ectopic pregnancy:

576. is associated with uterine enlargement.

577. is situated in the ovary in 5% of cases.

578. is more dangerous if situated in the cornual portion of the Fallopian tube.

579. commonly results in broad ligament haematoma.

580. may coexist with intrauterine pregnancy.

Tubal patency may be properly demonstrated by:

581. hysterosalpingography.

582. air insufflation.

583. laparoscopy and dye.

584. selective salpingography.

585. hysteroscopy.

The following are recognized complications of treatment of anovulatory infertility:

586. multiple pregnancy.

587. ectopic pregnancy.

588. cervical mucus hostility.

589. postural hypotension.

590. ascites.

Dilatation and curettage:

591. should be carried out in all patients with menorrhagia.

592. should be carried out in all patients with irregular bleeding.

593. should be recommended for all patients with break through bleeding on the combined oral contraceptive pill.

594. is an essential investigation for infertility.

595. may be helpful in the diagnosis of ectopic pregnancy.

The following are recognized complications of termination of pregnancy using prostaglandins:

596. utero-vaginal fistula.

597. pyrexia.

598. bronchospasm.

599. rupture of the uterus.

600. hyponatraemia.

MCQ ANSWERS
The answers, if true (T) or false (F), are given below:

1. F	15. F	29. F	43. T
2. T	16. T	30. T	44. F
3. T	17. F	31. T	45. F
4. F	18. F	32. T	46. T
5. F	19. T	33. F	47. T
6. T	20. T	34. F	48. F
7. F	21. F	35. T	49. F
8. T	22. F	36. T	50. T
9. T	23. F	37. T	51. F
10. T	24. T	38. T	52. F
11. T	25. T	39. T	53. T
12. F	26. T	40. T	54. F
13. T	27. T	41. F	55. F
14. F	28. T	42. T	56. T

57. F	97. F	137. T	177. T
58. T	98. F	138. T	178. T
59. T	99. F	139. T	179. F
60. F	100. F	140. T	180. T
61. T	101. T	141. T	181. T
62. T	102. F	142. T	182. F
63. F	103. T	143. F	183. F
64. F	104. F	144. T	184. F
65. T	105. T	145. F	185. F
66. F	106. T	146. F	186. F
67. T	107. F	147. T	187. T
68. T	108. T	148. T	188. T
69. F	109. F	149. T	189. T
70. F	110. F	150. F	190. T
71. F	111. T	151. T	191. T
72. F	112. T	152. T	192. F
73. T	113. T	153. F	193. T
74. F	114. T	154. F	194. T
75. T	115. T	155. T	195. T
76. T	116. F	156. F	196. T
77. T	117. F	157. F	197. F
78. F	118. T	158. F	198. T
79. F	119. T	159. T	199. T
80. T	120. T	160. T	200. T
81. T	121. T	161. T	201. F
82. T	122. T	162. F	202. T
83. T	123. T	163. T	203. T
84. F	124. F	164. T	204. T
85. F	125. F	165. T	205. F
86. T	126. T	166. F	206. T
87. T	127. T	167. T	207. T
88. F	128. T	168. T	208. F
89. T	129. T	169. F	209. F
90. T	130. T	170. F	210. F
91. F	131. T	171. T	211. F
92. T	132. F	172. T	212. F
93. F	133. F	173. F	213. F
94. F	134. F	174. F	214. F
95. T	135. F	175. T	215. T
96. T	136. F	176. F	216. F

217. F	257. T	297. F	337. F
218. T	258. T	298. F	338. T
219. F	259. F	299. F	339. T
220. T	260. F	300. T	340. F
221. T	261. T	301. T	341. F
222. F	262. T	302. F	342. T
223. T	263. T	303. F	343. T
224. T	264. F	304. T	344. T
225. T	265. F	305. T	345. F
226. T	266. F	306. F	346. T
227. T	267. F	307. F	347. T
228. T	268. T	308. T	348. T
229. T	269. T	309. F	349. T
230. T	270. F	310. T	350. T
231. T	271. T	311. T	351. F
232. T	272. T	312. F	352. T
233. T	273. F	313. F	353. T
234. T	274. T	314. F	354. T
235. F	275. T	315. T	355. F
236. T	276. T	316. T	356. T
237. F	277. T	317. F	357. F
238. T	278. F	318. T	358. F
239. T	279. T	319. T	359. F
240. F	280. F	320. T	360. T
241. T	281. T	321. F	361. T
242. T	282. T	322. F	362. T
243. F	283. F	323. T	363. F
244. T	284. T	324. F	364. T
245. T	285. F	325. F	365. T
246. T	286. T	326. T	366. T
247. F	287. T	327. F	367. F
248. F	288. T	328. F	368. T
249. T	289. F	329. T	369. T
250. F	290. T	330. T	370. T
251. F	291. F	331. F	371. T
252. T	292. F	332. F	372. T
253. F	293. T	333. F	373. F
254. F	294. T	334. T	374. T
255. T	295. F	335. T	375. T
256. T	296. T	336. F	376. F

377. F	417. T	457. F	497. T
378. T	418. T	458. T	498. T
379. F	419. T	459. F	499. T
380. F	420. F	460. T	500. T
381. T	421. T	461. T	501. F
382. T	422. T	462. T	502. T
383. T	423. T	463. T	503. T
384. T	424. F	464. F	504. T
385. T	425. T	465. T	505. T
386. F	426. T	466. T	506. T
387. T	427. T	467. T	507. F
388. T	428. T	468. T	508. F
389. T	429. F	469. F	509. T
390. F	430. F	470. F	510. T
391. T	431. F	471. F	511. F
392. F	432. F	472. T	512. T
393. F	433. T	473. T	513. F
394. F	434. F	474. T	514. T
395. T	435. T	475. T	515. T
396. F	436. F	476. F	516. T
397. F	437. T	477. T	517. F
398. T	438. T	478. T	518. T
399. T	439. F	479. F	519. F
400. T	440. F	480. T	520. T
401. T	441. F	481. F	521. F
402. T	442. T	482. T	522. F
403. T	443. F	483. T	523. F
404. F	444. F	484. F	524. T
405. F	445. F	485. T	525. F
406. F	446. F	486. F	526. F
407. T	447. F	487. T	527. T
408. T	448. T	488. F	528. T
409. F	449. F	489. F	529. T
410. T	450. T	490. T	530. T
411. T	451. F	491. F	531. F
412. T	452. F	492. T	532. T
413. T	453. T	493. T	533. T
414. T	454. T	494. F	534. T
415. F	455. T	495. T	535. T
416. F	456. T	496. T	536. F

537. F	553. T	569. F	585. F
538. T	554. T	570. T	586. T
539. T	555. F	571. F	587. F
540. T	556. F	572. F	588. T
541. T	557. F	573. T	589. T
542. T	558. T	574. T	590. T
543. T	559. T	575. F	591. F
544. T	560. T	576. T	592. F
545. T	561. T	577. F	593. F
546. T	562. F	578. T	594. F
547. F	563. F	579. F	595. T
548. T	564. F	580. T	596. T
549. T	565. T	581. T	597. T
550. F	566. T	582. F	598. T
551. F	567. F	583. T	599. T
552. T	568. F	584. T	600. F

12

Essay Questions

Introduction

The written examination in the Part 2 MRCOG contains two essay papers. The first paper, lasting 2 hours, consists of five short answer essay questions primarily concerning obstetrics and those relevant aspects of medicine, surgery, paediatrics and gynaecology. The second paper, also lasting 2 hours, consists of five short answer essay questions primarily concerning gynaecology and those relevant aspects of medicine, surgery and obstetrics.

Importance of the essays

Essay questions form two-thirds of the written paper, which is by far the most important part of the Part 2 examination; only candidates who pass the written can proceed to the oral assessment examination. Thus, the essays could be regarded as holding the key to the whole examination. A poor performance in the essays can not usually be compensated for by a good performance in the MCQ and will most probably result in failure in the written paper and, consequently, in the whole examination. Indeed, the RCOG has repeatedly identified this as a problem area and the main cause of failure in the Part 2 examination (in the March 1999 exam 81% of candidates failed the written paper). The importance of adequate preparation for the essays cannot be over emphasized.

Adequate preparation

Candidates usually believe that when they have read a chapter about, say, menstrual disorders, they are well prepared to answer any essay about that subject. The candidate probably thinks: 'I have read thoroughly about menstrual disorders and I understand the subject well. I can properly manage patients presenting with this complaint, so surely I should be able to answer related essays in the examination'.

This, in fact, is a common misconception and a sense of false security felt by many candidates. To illustrate the point further, let us imagine that you are sitting an examination that tests your skills in *performing* Caesarean section (CS). To prepare properly you do not just *read* about how to perform CS, but you also *perform* the procedure as many times as it takes you to be confident that you will do it properly in the examination. Your practice should also be under critical supervision, so mistakes could be identified and corrected before – rather than during – the examination. The same should apply to your preparation for the Part 2 MRCOG. It is testing your skill in *writing* essays; you should practice by *writing* essays.

Practice is even more important with this type of 'short answer' essays currently used in the MRCOG. Most candidates associate essay questions with spending about 1 hour writing many pages in the answer. This was correct with the previously used 'long answer' essay questions. The current examination system, however, allows only about 20 minutes or so for each answer and requires no more than two sides of A4 page. Prior practice is essential here to be able to concentrate your thoughts and write down the relevant points in this relatively limited time and space.

When to start

It is suggested that you should start practising at least 6 months before the date of your examination. You should aim to write five essays every week, so by the end of the 6 months you would have covered over 100 different subjects. This might sound a lot of work, but in practice it means only 2 hours of essay writing every week; a very reasonable investment towards maximizing your chances of success.

An alternative suggestion might be to start practising 3 months before the examination and answer 10 essays every week. However, it might be very difficult to find someone to mark 10 essays every week. Essay marking is a time consuming task, and your seniors will be more willing to do it whole-heartedly if given fewer essays per week.

Supervising your preparation

Seniors
Critical supervision is essential for adequate preparation, so faults can be identified and corrected aiming for a polished performance in the

examination. You should aim to have most of your practice essays marked by your seniors (Consultants and Senior Registrars). As they have been in a similar position in the past, they understand your needs. If approached at the right time and asked politely, they are unlikely to refuse. You should ask as many of them as possible to reduce the burden on each one. In addition, you will gain different valuable tips and ideas from each one, thus maximizing your benefit from the whole exercise.

Practice Groups

A number of candidates who are sitting the Part 2 examination at the same time can arrange an 'essay practice' group. Each candidate could answer a different essay at home. This, presented in front of the group, would increase the number of topics covered collectively and be of benefit to all participants. It will also mean that when your morale is low and affecting your motivation (not an uncommon occurrence prior to examinations), the motivation of the others will carry you through.

We suggest that you meet for 2–3 hours, once every 2 weeks at a time convenient for everybody to attend. The local postgraduate centre or medical library might be an ideal place. The secretary/librarian is usually very helpful in arranging after-hours attendance or an isolated meeting room. Participants do not necessarily have to be from the same hospital. If you approach obstetric and gynaecological trainees in neighbouring hospitals, you will be amazed by their favourable response. In fact, you will be doing them a great favour by arranging these groups. We have found that this is one of the best methods of essay practice. It bears all the hallmarks of successful preparation; a lot of practice, critical supervision and continuous motivation.

Courses

Most MRCOG Part 2 courses have special sessions for essay preparation and practice. These are usually very useful as they are run by experienced tutors who give valuable guidance. However, due to the limited time in any course, understandably there is no time for adequate practice. Appendix 2 provides details of suitable courses.

The question

Source of Questions

Previous examinations essay questions are very occasionally repeated, and it could be said that almost all the subjects that you could be asked about have already appeared in previous examinations. At the end of this chapter there is a collection of example questions.

The Element of Surprise

One of the main reasons why examinations are very testing and nerve wrecking is that you do not know what questions you will be asked. For your practice to be of real value, you should reproduce this element; you do not know what question you are going to answer until you sit down, pen and paper ready and the clock starts ticking away. A friend or a member of your family can randomly select a question from a large collection and read it out for you, just before you answer it. Alternatively, one of your colleagues can write the question on a paper and fold it for you to unfold immediately before you start answering. This is because there is no point in knowing what question you are going to attempt hours or days in advance. Invariably you will be thinking of it and preparing the answer in your mind. This luxury is, unfortunately, not available in the real examination. The same applies to reading a chapter about a particular subject then answering a related essay. It defeats the whole object of the exercise, which is to reproduce the examination situation as much as possible.

Types of Questions

Basically, there are two main types of essay questions, each requiring a different approach in the answer:

1. The first type is the 'Discuss/ Critically evaluate/ Critically appraise/ Debate...' question. Examples are:

   Discuss the use of anticoagulant drugs in obstetrics.
   Hysterectomy for dysfunctional uterine bleeding is out of date. Discuss.
   Critically appraise the use of the colposcope in gynaecological practice.

   When answering this type of question, you should imagine that you are the learned expert giving a lecture to post-Membership doctors or writing an editorial about the subject in a medical journal. In fact, editorials and commentaries in journals are very good illustrations of how these questions should be answered. They start by briefly outlining the condition and its importance (e.g. incidence, effect on maternal/perinatal mortality/ morbidity), then go on to dedicate the main bulk of the essay to presenting a critical account of the predisposing factors, aetiology, presentation, symptoms, signs, special investigations, differential diagnosis, prevention, treatment, follow-up and so as appropriate. Controversial issues are explored in depth, and the pros and cons of different options are discussed before reaching a reasoned conclusion.

2. The second type is the 'clinical situation' essay. Theoretically it is the easiest to answer as it asks candidates to write about what they do in every day clinical practice. Examples include:

A 19-year-old woman attends the gynaecological clinic because she has not menstruated for 1year. Discuss your management .
Describe the management of a woman with infertility and oligomenorrhoea.
Discuss the management of a patient with fulminating pre-eclampsia.

The best way to answer this type of question is to reflect on your clinical practice and write what you would do, and why, if confronted with such a clinical situation. This will almost always be in the format of presentation, history, examination, investigations, treatment and follow-up.

The answer

In the examination you are given an answer booklet, with two sides of lined A4 available for the answer of each essay.

First, Read the Question

This is the commonest advice given in any examination. Yet, it is the least followed. The number of MRCOG candidates that misread words like 'infertility' as 'fertility', 'pre-eclampsia' as 'eclampsia' or write extensively about the past obstetric history in answering a question about a primigravida, makes repeating this advice very valid. Read the question *twice*, then underline the *key points* as these will tell you what type of question it is and what exactly it is asking for. The following example should illustrate this point:

Discuss the use of *anticoagulant drugs* in *obstetrics*.

So the three key points are: *Discuss* (a critical evaluation-type question), *anticoagulant drugs* (main subject) and *obstetrics* (so do not mention anticoagulants in radical pelvic surgery or prophylaxis in gynaecological operations).

Anatomy of the Essay

1. Plan
   This is the vertebral column of the answer on which you can attach other parts and build a complete essay. Having read the question *twice*, underlined the key points and understood what is required, you should now spend about 2 minutes planning the general structure of the answer.

The skill is in deciding on the most important points to include *before* you start writing down the answer. This is particularly important because you have a relatively short time to answer each question (five essays in 2 hours). If you do not plan your answer in advance, you may spend a long time discussing an important point, only to discover that there is another equally important point that deserves discussion, but with no time available. The instructions to Examiners (see later) indicate specific marks for each point, and elaboration on one point will not compensate for omission of another. Although the plan is not written down and is not marked, nevertheless, it helps you to organize your thoughts and makes essay writing a straightforward process.

2. Introduction

   This is the first brief paragraph of the 'Discuss/ Evaluate/ Critically appraise/ Debate' type of essays, where you give a broad overview of the subject and what you intend to discuss in the main body. You also show the Examiner that you understand the importance of the subject in question. This should be in the form of factual information. For example, when answering a question about thromboembolism or anticoagulant drugs, it is very pertinent to introduce your essay by mentioning that thromboembolism is one of the commonest causes of maternal mortality in the UK. Similarly, in answering a question about infertility you should mention that it affects 1 in 6 couples. Percentages and figures are the most powerful tools of illustrating factual information, and you are well advised to learn those related to common conditions. Important points include: effects on perinatal/ maternal mortality/ morbidity, incidence, 5-year survival rates and cost-effectiveness.

3. Body of the essay

   This consists of a number of paragraphs, each discussing a distinct issue related to the subject. Emphasis on the discussion is very important, as at the Membership level simple listing and enumeration is neither adequate nor acceptable. What is required is a mature discussion reflecting your understanding of the controversial issues and leading to a reasoned conclusion.

4. Conclusion

   This is the final paragraph in the essay. It includes a *resumé* of the essential points and important arguments, together with your own conclusions and the reasons behind them. As this is the part the Examiner reads last before deciding your mark, it should be positively strong. A good essay which ends abruptly without a conclusion (most probably because the candidate has run out of time) is unlikely to attract the usual discretionary marks.

Handwriting and Presentation

It goes with out saying that the Examiners cannot mark what they cannot read. It is of primary importance that you should write legibly. Many people think that they can never improve their handwriting, but this is not true. Legible handwriting is a skill, not a talent, and it is learned by practice. Practice makes perfect, or at least makes legible. You need to practice writing larger, clearly and slowly. Some suggest writing with a 'fluid-ink' pen as this will make you write slowly. You have to make sure, however, that you do not smudge the ink on the paper, which is easily done with these pens. The best advice is to try different types of pens during your practice until you find the one that suits you most and makes your writing clearer.

You also have to make sure that your answer is tidy, with not much crossing out. If you make a mistake, it is better to use a single line to cross it (e.g. ~~labor~~) as this will appear more tidy than using multiple heavy lines. The best thing, of course, is to avoid crossing all together.

A good tip, next to being perfect and making no mistakes, is to use correction fluid (e.g. Tipp-Ex) to cover any mistake. Several brands are available in the market, and you are well advised to try some of them during your practice and decide on the most appropriate one to take to the examination.

To aid the clarity of the answer, it is worth writing headings for the main paragraphs and underlining the key words using a different colour (e.g. red). Do remember to take a ruler to the examination as zig-zag lines are not very presentable.

Timing the Answer

One of the main aspects of examinations in general is the limited time available for answering. In the Part 2 written examination you are given 2 hours to answer five essay questions, and you should dedicate about 20–25 minutes for each question. Many candidates, having found that they know more about one or more questions than the rest (which is not unusual), spend most of the time answering those questions at the expense of the others. This is based on the mistaken belief that an excellent answer will compensate for a very poor one.

The first 2 minutes should be dedicated to the plan, the following 20 minutes to the actual essay, and the last 2 minutes to revision and corrections. This revision is very important as the absence or presence of small words like 'not' can make a big difference to the meaning. What you can write in 20 minutes, you can say in 3–4 minutes depending on your speed. It might appear unfair that you are expected to write an essay about a big subject like preterm labour in such a short space of time. It is the purpose of the examination, however, to test your ability in presenting the important and relevant information in the allocated time.

You should start your practice by answering one question in 25 minutes. As you get more practice, you should be given more questions in more time, aiming for five questions in 2 hours, just like the real exam. Many candidates, having practised only with one question at a time, find it difficult to concentrate while answering the rest of the questions in the real examination.

Good English

Your aim is to convey your scientific thoughts clearly and concisely using good English language. This is best achieved by dividing your essay into paragraphs each addressing a separate issue. Short sentences, each containing no more than two clauses and presenting a single clear idea are easier to construct and understand than complex multi-claused sentences. Thoughts should flow logically and effortlessly from one sentence to the next. Connecting words such as 'however, nevertheless, therefore, in addition, furthermore, on the other hand' should be used accordingly. The third person should be used in preference to the first person. Abbreviations should be written in full when first mentioned. Editorials in medical journals are very good examples of scientific English. The more editorials you read, the closer your own style will get to them.

Examiners' instructions

For each essay, the Examiners are given a structured marking scheme with suggested guidelines on how many marks to be allocated to each part of the answer. Half marks may be used for components within the answers but the total must be rounded *down* to a whole mark. For each answer, 2 marks are allocated for logical coherent expression and overall impression. One or both of these marks may be lost for serious factual errors.

Example questions and Examiners' instructions

Two exam papers (10 questions) are give below, together with their Examiners' instructions.

Paper 1

Question 1
Describe the pre-conceptual counselling that you would offer a 25-year-old nulliparous woman whose natural father suffers from haemophilia A (Factor VIII deficiency).

Examiners' Instructions

Concept:
The candidate understands that haemophilia is a sex-linked recessive disorder and that the woman is an obligate carrier.   **1 Mark**

A good candidate should:

- Determine that the woman and her partner understand the implication of the inheritance:
  a. 50% of male offspring will have haemophilia and 50% of the female offspring will have carrier status.   **1 Mark**
  b. the woman herself may have a very low level of Factor VIII putting her at risk of excessive haemorrhage at delivery.   **1 Mark**

- Discuss methods of determining the sex of the fetus: **2 Marks**
  a. C.V.S. at 8–12 weeks, and its problems.
  b. amniocentesis and its problems.
  c. ultrasound examination.
  d. cordocentesis.

- Discuss accurate diagnosis by DNA sampling.   **1 Mark**

- Explain that preselection of gender is not possible.   **1 Mark**

- Determine the couple's attitude towards a male fetus, especially if it was found to be affected.   **1 Mark**
  Discretionary points.   **2 Marks**

  Total Mark   10

Question 2
Debate the need for antenatal beds in an obstetric unit.

Examiners' Instructions
A good candidate should:

- Know that most patients traditionally managed antenatally as in-patients could be cared for adequately in home environment, *BUT* must accept that certain categories have to be managed in hospital.   **1 Mark**

- Critically appraise the need for patients with IUGR, hypertension, PPROM, etc. to be in hospital.   **1 Mark**

- Discuss: **4 Marks**
  a. the management of medical disorders in pregnancy.
  b. the place of Day Units, out-patient biophysical profiles, CTG, blood tests, etc.
  c. the role of the community midwife and GP.
  d. the geographical location of the unit in relation to the patient's home and the domestic circumstances, living conditions, etc.
  e. use of gynaecology wards for some disorders, e.g. hyperemesis and midtrimester bleeding.

- Understand the consequences, such as: **2 Marks**
  a. financial implications.
  b. compliance of patient.
  c. education of midwife and GP.

Discretionary points.   **2 Marks**

Total Mark   10

Question 3
A 27-year-old woman who has recently undergone renal transplantation is contemplating pregnancy. What advice, specific to her condition, would you give her?

Examiners' Instructions
A good candidate would be expected to know:

- That if the reason for renal failure was a familiar disorder, e.g. polycystic kidney disease, genetic counselling should be offered.   **1 Mark**

- The importance of various drugs: **2 Marks**
  A. high dose steroids – the risks of teratogenic effects.
  B. immuno-suppressants – be aware that there are no
     reported problems.
  C. antihypertensives – change from ACE inhibitors and
     pure beta-blockers.
  D. antibiotics - continue though a change of drug may
     be necessary.

- That there is an increased risk of pregnancy induced
  hypertension.   **1 Mark**

- That there should be regular assessments of renal function
  (urea/urate/creatinine). Be aware that pregnancy does not
  adversely affect renal function.   **1 Mark**

- That there is an increased risk of early and late pregnancy
  loss. Advise regular assessment of fetal growth.   **1 Mark**

- That the timing and mode of delivery (e.g. Caesarean
  section) depend upon obstetric factors only.   **1 Mark**

- That a transplanted kidney does not obstruct labour.   **1 Mark**

Discretionary points.   **2 Marks**

                                   Total Mark   10

Question 4

Evaluate treatments available in the management of a patient with severe pre-eclampsia in the 32nd week of her first pregnancy.

Examiners' Instructions

A good candidate would be expected to know:

- That the definitive treatment is delivery but that this may
  need to be delayed in balancing prematurity against
  maternal risk.   **1 Mark**

- About the use of corticosteroids for prophylaxis against
  respiratory distress syndrome (RDS).   **1 Mark**

- About the choice of different antihypertensive agents,
  including justification for their use in this case.   **1 Mark**

- About the prevention and treatment of convulsions
  (magnesium sulphate the treatment of choice).   **2 Marks**

- About the importance of fluid balance.   **1 Mark**

- About the timing and mode of delivery.   **1 Mark**

- When to involve other specialities or other units.   **1 Mark**

Discretionary points.   **2 Marks**

Total Mark   10

Question 5

A nulliparous 28-year-old woman presents at 8 weeks' gestation with uterine bleeding. An ultrasound scan reveals a viable pregnancy in one horn of a bicornuate uterus. How would you advise her?

Examiners' Instructions

A good candidate should:

- Be able to explain a possible range of outcomes in early
  pregnancy from a threatened miscarriage with reassurance
  to uterine rupture, depending upon the details of the uterine
  malformation itself.   **2 Marks**

- Explain the nature of the abnormality to the patient.   **1 Mark**

- Explain the range of outcomes in late pregnancy, including
  normality, preterm labour, malpresentations, cord prolapse,
  intrauterine growth restriction and the possible need for
  Caesarean section.   **3 Marks**

- Explain the need for increased antenatal surveillance.   **1 Mark**

- Give advice for the future management, including the
  exclusion of associated renal tract abnormalities.   **1 Mark**

- Discretionary points.   **2 Marks**

Total Mark   10

Paper 2

Question 6

A 40-year-old woman with a uterus enlarged by fibroids and with normal cervical cytology, is advised to have an abdominal hysterectomy. Explain the potential benefits and disadvantages of the sub-total operation.

Examiners' Instructions
A good candidate should:

- Know of decreased risk of primary haemorrhage and damage to surrounding organs such as ureters, bladder, etc.   **1 Mark**

- Know of decreased morbidity regarding secondary haemorrhage, infection, bladder dysfunction, vault granulations.   **2 Marks**

- Be aware of shorter anaesthetic and operating time.   **1 Mark**

- Know that patient can resume sexual intercourse earlier and that (possibly) there will be better vaginal lubrication.   **1 Mark**

- Know of the need of continuing cervical cytology and be aware that cervical pathology could arise in the future.   **1 Mark**

- Know that menstruation may resume from endometrial remnants in the cervical canal.   **1 Mark**

- Know the importance of providing explanatory leaflets and record risk/benefits discussed with the patient in the notes.   **1 Mark**

- Discretionary points.   **2 Marks**

Total Mark   10

Question 7
Summarize the causes and management of severe ovarian hyperstimulation syndrome.

Examiners' Instructions
This question explores that the candidates has knowledge of the risks of stimulation with HMG, understands the grading of OHSS and recognizes that severe OHSS is life threatening

- *A good candidate would be expected to know that:*   **2 Marks**
  a. the condition is iatrogenic resulting from supra physiological stimulation of the ovaries in the course of ovulation induction (conception is not a pre-requisite).

    b. the key features are ovarian enlargement due to multiple cysts associated with increased capillary permeability, leading to fluid shifts out of the intravascular space.

    c. symptoms are related to acute painful enlargement of the ovaries, depletion of the intravascular volume, hyponatraemia and complications arising from the effusions.

- Investigations should include FBC, urea and electrolytes, creatinine, liver function tests, coagulation profile, ultrasound scanning and CXR. **2 Marks**

- Vital signs and urine output should be monitored, with correction of intravascular volume (i.v. fluids, albumin and the use of CVP line). **1 Mark**

- Drainage of effusions may be required. **1 Mark**

- Thromboprophylaxis (including heparin) is essential, **1 Mark**

- Admission to an ITU may be necessary, surgical drainage of cysts on rare occasions, exceptionally termination of pregnancy. **1 Mark**

- Discretionary points. **2 Marks**

                                      Total Mark　10

Question 8

A 36-year-old patient with many years of primary subfertility becomes pregnant spontaneously. At referral to a consultant antenatal clinic, it is reported that her most recent cervical cytology shows severe dyskaryosis. Colposcopy is carried out at 14 weeks' gestation and diathermy loop excision of the lesion is carried out, can you justify her management?

Examiners' Instructions

A good candidate should:

- Know the natural history of CIN 3 and recognize that only about 30% will develop invasion in the next 20 years. **2 Marks**

- Know that colposcopy is essential to make a diagnosis and to exclude overt invasion. **1 Mark**

- Understand that the relationship between cytology, colposcopic findings and histology is a poor one. **1 Mark**

- Recognize the risks of haemorrhage, infection and the perception of miscarriage. **2 Marks**

- Understand the alternative, i.e. regular colposcopic examination without biopsy throughout pregnancy. **1 Mark**

- Counsel the patient accordingly, explaining both the advantages and risks of the course that she would take. **1 Mark**

- Discretionary points. **2 Marks**

Total Mark 10

Question 9

A 30-year-old nulliparous woman presents with severe dysmenorrhoea and dyspareunia. Laparoscopy confirms bilateral ovarian endometriomata, 5 cm in diameter and adhesive disease to the rectum. She has been using barrier contraception but is planning pregnancy in a year's time. Briefly debate the use of gonadotrophin-releasing hormone analogues (GnRH-a).

Examiners' Instructions

A good candidate should be expected:

- To understand the rationale and routes of GnRH-a administration. **2 Marks**

- To appreciate that the side-effects of GnRH-a compared to other treatments are more acceptable to the patient. **2 Marks**

- To know that it offers an opportunity to perform surgery on endometriomata > 3 cm whilst on treatment. **1 Mark**

- To know that relapse will occur in time whatever treatment is given. **1 Mark**

- To be aware of the higher cost. **1 Mark**

- To advise patients of a window of opportunity for conception and/or the place of IVF therapy following treatment. **1 Mark**

Discretionary points. **2 Marks**

Total Mark 10

Question 10

A 53-year-old woman undergoes total abdominal hysterectomy and bilateral salpingo-oophorectomy for a stage lB endometrial cancer. Evaluate the risks and benefits of hormone replacement therapy (HRT) for her.

Examiners' Instructions

The candidate should address the use of HRT in any woman of this age and the quality of her life. He/she should consider whether oestrogens with or without progestogens should be used in patients with an oestrogen-sensitive tumour.

A good candidate should know:

- That there is no evidence that a patient with a very early tumour, as in this case, is likely to have an increased risk of recurrence with HRT.   **1 Mark**

- That systemic oestrogens are the only reliable treatment for severe vasomotor symptoms. Topical oestrogens for vaginal symptoms should be considered.   **1 Mark**

- That long-term oestrogen therapy protects against osteoporosis and may protect against cardiovascular and Alzheimer's disease, but that there are no completed prospective randomized trials to confirm the cardiovascular benefits.   **2 Marks**

- That an increase in collagen affecting skin, ligaments, bone etc. will occur with HRT, and that enhancement of libido and mood may occur.   **1 Mark**

- That the risks include an increased incidence of breast cancer after 8 years, of venous thrombosis and a perception of weight gain etc.   **2 Marks**

- That the combination of a progestogen if HRT is given systemically is possibly of use but that progestogens given alone are of no proven benefit.   **1 Mark**

Discretionary points.   **2 Marks**

Total Mark   10

Example question

For your own practice, another 10 questions are given below. Each five should be considered as a separate exam paper and attempted in 2 hours.

1. Critically evaluate the methods available for detecting diabetes mellitus in pregnancy.

2. Justify your management of a 30-year-old primigravid woman who attends the antenatal clinic at 33 weeks' gestation with a blood pressure of 140 over 100 mmHg and 2 ++ proteinuria. Her pregnancy was previously uncomplicated.

3. A 30-year-old primigravid woman requests amniocentesis to exclude Down's syndrome. How would you counsel her?

4. Describe the use of mifepristone (RU486) in first trimester termination of pregnancy. What other potential uses does this drug have in obstetrics and gynaecology?

5. Evaluate the role of ultrasound scanning in multiple pregnancies.

6. Critically evaluate the role of qualitative beta HCG assays in the management of early pregnancy problems.

7. Discuss the investigation and treatment of a man with azoospermia.

8. Discuss the assessment of a woman with chronic pelvic pain.

9. Critically evaluate the role of laparoscopy in the management of ectopic pregnancy.

10. A 52-year-old woman taking HRT is concerned about recent reports about increased risk of venous thromboembolism. How would you counsel her?

KEY POINTS

- The essay questions form two-thirds of the written paper which must be passed before a candidate is allowed to complete the Part 2 examination. Poor performance in the essays is frequently identified as the main cause of failure.

- Adequate preparation implies practising essay writing in circumstances similar to the real examination. These include: not knowing the question in advance, answering five essays in 2 hours, and getting your answers marked.

- Legible handwriting, good English and coherent answers are as important as factual knowledge.

13

The Oral Assessment Examination

Introduction

The results of the written paper will be posted to you approximately 4 weeks after the examination. Candidates who obtain the pass mark (175 out of 300) or above are invited to attend the oral assessment examination. This takes place approximately 10 weeks after the written paper, during the second/third week in May and November (for the March and September examinations, respectively), and is held in the UK (London) and occasionally in some overseas centres (e.g. Hong Kong for the 1999 examination). In this chapter we will discuss the oral assessment examination; its evolution, importance, format, scope, types of questions asked and how to prepare for each type.

Evolution of the oral assessment examination

From November 1998 the oral assessment examination replaced the clinical and viva (oral) examinations in the Part 2 MRCOG. There was a perceived unfairness of the format of those examinations. Too many variables had been introduced by the examination system itself and in consequence it was neither fair nor valid. The problem was further complicated by difficulty in recruiting suitable patients who were now less willing to participate in clinical examinations and, in particular, less willing to be clinically examined.

The new oral assessment examination is designed to expose candidates to a greater number of Examiners and consequently to reduce the effect of any one Examiner on the candidate's score. Each candidate will be tested on the same topics as his or her peers.

Importance of the oral assessment examination

Candidates and Examiners alike often complain that examinations are artificial; they test candidates in tasks (e.g. essay writing, MCQ) that do not form part of their normal daily clinical work. In this sense the oral assessment examination is the most fair and real part of the MRCOG examination. It tests candidates in what they have been doing for years on a day-to-day basis: taking clinical histories, talking to 'patients' and formulating management plans. A polished performance is, therefore, expected and mistakes are less likely to be excused. The required standards are high but no higher than those expected from you in everyday practice.

The importance the RCOG places on the oral assessment examination is clearly illustrated in the marking system. However high your mark in the written paper is, you *must* pass the oral assessment examination (i.e. score at least 60 out of 100) in order to pass the Part 2 MRCOG.

Format of the oral assessment examination

This consists of an assessment circuit containing 12 stations. Ten of these stations will be 'active' and have an Examiner present, and two stations will be 'preparatory' for the following station. Each station is 15 minutes long and at some stage during the examination there will be a 10-minute break for candidates and Examiners to rest and use cloakroom facilities if necessary. You will be assigned a starting station and a circuit on a particular day, and when the bell rings you move on to the following station, and so on. The total length of the examination lasts for 3 hours and 10 minutes. The format of the examination will be identical on all 3 days of the examination, but the actual questions will be different.

There are no real patients in the exam, but some active stations will have a 'role-player' in addition to the Examiner. These role-players are trained actors and actresses. In the exam they take the role of a patient or a relative, depicting a particular scenario in order to assess your communication skills. In some stations, the Examiner him/herself will act as the role-player.

Examiners at each station are given general instructions about the marking scheme and how many marks to be allocated to each part of the answer. These are for guidance only and are there to ensure consistency in marking – as much as possible. The Examiners have the latitude to explore in depth a candidate's knowledge and understanding.

Scope of the oral examination

The Examiners can ask about virtually anything to do with obstetrics and gynaecology. However, the expected depth of your answer and how it is assessed will vary according to the question asked. As we have discussed previously, the Membership examination is aimed at obstetric and gynaecological Specialist Registrars in the UK and their equivalents. The knowledge expected from you is similar to what you are expected to know as a Specialist Registrar. This includes detailed management of common clinical problems as well as basic management of the less common conditions. In addition to your factual knowledge, the Examiners will be assessing your ability of reasoning and deduction as well as your communication skills.

Points to ponder

Your aim in the oral assessment examination is to demonstrate your knowledge, common sense, analytical thinking and communication skills. The following points are worth noting as you go into the examination. All of us forget some of these points at sometime or another.

1. Appearance:
   Your Examiners will see you before hearing your answers. If you appear like a professional, they will perceive you as one. Professional appearance is equated with tidy hair, neat clothes and clean shoes.

2. Understand the question:
   Listen carefully and understand the question clearly. If you do not understand it, do not simply ask the Examiner to repeat it, as he (or she) will just do that; repeat it. Say that you do not understand the question, and the Examiner will rephrase it.

3. Engage mind before mouth:
   Many candidates are understandably anxious which tends to make them speak very quickly, often before thinking. This should be avoided at all costs, as it is very difficult to retract what you have just said. Always think before you answer. The Examiners permit, and indeed expect, you to think for a couple of seconds before you answer.

4. Answer the question you are asked:
   As we have seen above, many different types of questions could be asked about the same subject. Some candidates, under the stress of the

examination, go at a tangent and answer something totally different from what has been asked. For example, when asked how you would do a cone biopsy, it is not appropriate to concentrate on the indications for cone biopsy. No matter how you dislike the question you have been asked, or think that you can do better on a different related question, you have to play the hand you are dealt and answer the question as it is.

5. Self-confidence:
You should exhibit a self-confident attitude; appear cool and calm; speak in a voice that is neither aggressively loud nor timidly low and with a pace that is neither too quick nor hesitantly slow; look the Examiner in eye when you are answering; and appear to believe in what you are saying. Contrary to popular belief, self-confidence is an acquired attribute which takes much practice.

6. Reaction to stress:
As a doctor, you are subjected to stressful situations all the time. The Examiners will be trying to assess your reaction to stress by asking you difficult questions to which there may be no clear answer. Remember that only good candidates are asked these questions. If in difficulty, reflect on your clinical practice and imagine that you are facing the same situation in a clinical context. Then describe what you would have done and this will be the right answer. This answer may contain '... and I would then refer the patient to a more senior colleague for advice'. There is no magic; just plain common sense.

7. Do not repeat the question:
Examiners find candidates who repeat the questions very irritating. Whether you do it out of habit, nervousness, or because you want to gain a few seconds to think, stop doing it.

8. Do not dig your own grave:
You have to be able to justify anything you say and explain all your proposed actions. Do not 'drop in' conditions that you know very little about. The Examiners might think that you are trying to lead them up that path and, in trying to help you, they may ask you about it.

9. Do not argue:
This is a time-honoured advice, but some candidates still manage to ignore it. You may think, or even know for definite that your Examiner is wrong in something he/she has said, but the examination is neither the time nor the place to say so.

The questions and how to prepare

You may be asked different forms of types of questions at different stations, each requiring a different form of answer. It is very important to understand what type of question you are being asked and to know how to formulate the answer. Too often, a candidate may concentrate on the subject in question and ignore the form of the question. This will result in an answer very different from what the Examiner had in mind.

The following are the common forms of questions asked in the oral assessment examination, together with advice on how to answer them. The examples given are actual MRCOG questions which appeared in previous examinations.

1. Operative questions

    You may be asked to describe an operation in detail which may include preoperative and postoperative discussions. This will usually be about common operations with which you should be familiar. This question is usually asked in the form of a clinical scenario. For example '*A primigravid woman in spontaneous labour at term has failure of progressive cervical dilatation for 6 hours in the first stage of labour. This did not respond to artificial rupture of membranes and oxytocin infusion. You have decided to perform a Caesarean section. Discuss with the consultant on call (the Examiner) your preoperative, intraoperative and postoperative procedures*'.

    The preparation for such question should be part of your standard training. For every operation you perform, or assist in, you should be aware of the pre-, intra-, and postoperative details. In addition, you should also be able to explain these to your colleagues. If you practice in this way, this question in the exam should be 'plain sailing'. This illustrates a very important point; the major bulk of your preparation for the Part 2 MRCOG is during the 2–3 clinical training years before the exam, not just the preceding 2–3 months.

2. Communication and counselling skills

    Your communication skills will be assessed by your interaction with a role player depicting a particular scenario. For example, you may be told that '*the role player has had an unexplained intrapartum still-born baby at term on that day. How would counsel her and explain further investigations and management?*' Alternatively, you may be told that '*the role player is the husband of a woman who has had an unexplained intrapartum still-born baby at term 6 weeks previously. How would counsel him, explain the investigations findings (with which you are provided) and further management?*' Other situations could be explaining abnormal smear result and abnormal antenatal screening tests results.

These communication skills questions should cause no difficulty for candidates who have been communicating with patients and colleagues for a minimum of 3 years before sitting the Part 2 examination. However, the well-recognized tension and pressure of the examination might make you forget a few important points. These include introducing yourself to the patient, putting her/him at ease, establishing appropriate eye contact (with the patient and not Examiner), listening attentively, explaining the condition without the use of medical jargon, following verbal and non-verbal clues, pausing for the patient to ask questions and introduce new issues, and adequately explaining the intended course of action. Finally, all communications with patients should end with the question 'is there anything you would like to ask me?' or something similar. In such communication stations your impression on the role-players is as important as on the Examiners. In fact, the role-players contribute to your mark by indicating whether they have gained confidence in you during that encounter and whether they would like to see you as their doctor again.

3. History-taking

Your history-taking skills will be assessed in some stations. The role-player will pause as a patient presenting with a complaint, a GP referral letter, or an emergency presentation. This could be in either obstetrics or gynaecology. '*This 24-year-old woman has vaginal discharge. Take a full history from her and explain your further management*', or you could be asked, '*this woman is 30 weeks pregnant and is presenting with lower abdominal pain. Take a full history from her and explain your further management*'.

History-taking is actually a part of your everyday work as a junior doctor, and a polished performance is expected from you in this type of question. The key to delivering such a performance is to adopt a methodical approach. You should start with the the history of presenting complaint; past obstetric, gynaecological, medical and surgical history; social history; family history and so on. Here again, your concentration should be on the role-payer, not the Examiner.

4. The 'management' question

This is a clinical question requiring a clinical answer. You may be presented with a clinical problem or given an investigation result and asked how you would manage it. '*How would you manage an 18-year-old girl presenting with primary amenorrhoea and a serum prolactin of 2200 IU/L*'.

Notice that the Examiner wants to know how *you* would manage these cases. Therefore, your answer must start with '*I* would....'. This will give the impression that you are answering from clinical experience, rather than from books alone. You should also answer along the traditional clinical lines of history, examination, investigation, etc. Your answer should be like: 'I would take a full history and perform an adequate examination. In the history I would want to know about ... . In the examination I would look for... and so on.

There may be different management options and you will be expected to discuss the arguments for and against each option. You should also indicate that, if faced with such a condition, which option you will choose and why. Just simply to 'sit on the fence' is not adequate. Similarly, to choose an option because 'my Consultant says so' is equally unacceptable. All the controversial topics discussed in the oral assessment examination are common clinical conditions which you should have met, read about and considered during your training.

5. Surgical instruments

   You may be given a surgical equipment and asked to describe or assemble it. For example, in a recent examination candidates were given a '*cystoscope*' and asked to assemble it. The main bulk of the station was the discussion with the Examiner about the uses of that instrument. Other instruments that you may be given include obstetric forceps, ventouse, laparoscope, hysteroscope, etc.

   Sometimes you may be given an instrument which you have never seen before. Think again. If you are still sure that you do not know what it is, then say so. The Examiners know that different instruments are used in different hospitals, and with your relatively limited experience at this stage you are not expected to recognize every instrument. The Examiners will then try and give you clues that may help you recognizing the instrument. For example, a candidate may be given Fallope rings, but having never used them before, does not recognize them. If the candidate says so, the Examiner may say that an alternative is Filshie clip, and then the candidate is on the right track. Remember that the main bulk of this station is the clinical discussion.

6. Questions about emergencies

   These are a must, and almost every candidate is asked about the management of one emergency at least in one form or another during the examination. '*How would you manage a patient with severe postpartum haemorrhage?*' *How would you manage a patient with eclampsia? How would you manage a patient with shoulder dystocia?*'

Your answer must be practical, precise and direct. You should also mention first things first; the sequence of your proposed actions is of vital importance. There is only a limited number of emergencies in obstetrics and gynaecology. You are advised to practice answering such questions about all of them in preparation for your examination. Please remember that neonatal resuscitation is an obstetric emergency. Moreover, it is a common question in the examination.

7. Clinical skills

You may be asked to demonstrate some clinical skills on special dummies in the exam, such as speculum insertion, insertion of the laparoscope and cardiopulmonary resuscitation. This will be followed by a related discussion.

You have been performing all these clinical skills during your clinical work. Candidates are often very good in how they do things. What they are not as good in, however, is why they do them that way. For every thing you do, logically, there should be a reason. The way to practice for this type of question is to think of everything you do at work, how you do it and why.

8. Audit

You may be asked to design and discuss a particular audit protocol. For example '*design an audit protocol for induction of labour in post-term pregnancy*'. This type of question will be given to you in a 'preparatory' station, where you are given 15 minutes to consider the issue and design the protocol before discussing it with the Examiner at the next station.

Some candidates often confuse 'research' and 'audit'. Basically, research aims at finding the right thing to do, i.e. is labour induction in post-term pregnancy better than expectant management? Audit, on the other hand, aims at finding out if the right thing (or what we believe to be the right thing) is being done. For example, if our policy is to induce labour at 42 weeks gestation (because we believe it to be the right thing), we can do an audit to find out if we are actually doing this. Therefore, in order to do an audit of a particular practice you should agree on a gold standard to which you compare your practice. You should then find ways of collecting reliable information about your practice. This information is analyzed and compared to the agreed gold standard. Reasons for non-agreement should be explored and addressed, and ways of improving practice (i.e. making it more like the gold standard) should be agreed and implemented. The audit cycle is then completed by re-auditing the same issue after a reasonable period of time.

9. Critical appraisal and discussion of a short document

    You may be asked to critically appraise a short document (such as a case report, audit report, guideline, patient information sheet, etc.). For example, you may be given a patient leaflet about endometriosis and asked to critically appraise it. This type of question will be given to you in a 'preparatory' station, where you are given 15 minutes to read the document and consider its contents before discussing with the Examiner at the following station.

    The key to critically appraising any item is to recognize what it is trying to achieve, and then methodically examining if it has done this properly. We have already discussed in the previous section what an *audit* should do and how. A *case report* should briefly describe an interesting case that illustrates a useful educational point, which is not within the realm of everyday knowledge or mainstream textbooks. It should also include some sort of review of previously published similar cases, with comment on how this case differs from them. *Guidelines* should address a specific important clinical situation, be clear and unambiguous, and based on the best available evidence. *Patient information leaflets* should be clear, written in lay-person terms with no medical jargon, and contain accurate factual information including benefits, risks, side-effects and limitations (as appropriate). Try to critically appraise some guidelines and patient information leaflets in your hospital using these guidelines. You will find that using a systematic approach really pays off.

    The next chapter is dedicated to literature appraisal, and describes in detail how to deal with these issues.

10. Clinical understanding and priority setting

    You may be given a scenario where you have a number of clinical cases with varying degrees of urgency and asked to prioritize and divide the work between yourself and a number of doctors working with you. For example, you may be shown a '*labour ward board*' which contains information on a number of patients. A patient may have a prolonged second stage with an occipito-lateral position and at '0' station, another one has a prolonged second stage as well with a direct occipito anterior position and '+2' station, and a third patient who needs IV access because she is in active labour and has had a previous Caesarean section. You are told that you have with you an experienced career SHO and a GP-trainee SHO. How would you divide the work and why? In this situation you would see the first patient yourself, and probably deliver her in theatre as a trial; send the career SHO to the second patient; and ask the GP-trainee to attend to the last patient. The Examiner will discuss with you the reasons behind your choices and may introduce some other clinical variables to see how you respond to them. You are faced by similar situations everyday in your clinical work. The best practice is to know the reasons behind any clinical action or choice you make.

11. The 'set topic' question

This is usually an open question about a particular subject, and is similar to the old style conventional oral examination. *'Tell me about hysteroscopy. Tell me about endometriosis'.* The Examiners are giving you an open invitation to display your knowledge about a topic which they expect you to know well.

This is a golden opportunity for you to show the breadth of your knowledge and you should deliver a polished performance. Your answer should be factual, organized and you should not appear as if you have never thought of this subject before.

12. Eponymous questions

An eponym is the name of a disease, structure, operation or procedure derived from the name of the person who discovered or described it first. Such questions are not infrequently asked in the oral assessment examination, not as a separate station but as a part of other stations. *'Who was Braxton-Hicks? Who was Kielland? Who was Doppler? Who was Pfannenstiel?'*

These questions should never be a cause for concern, as they are almost always asked of good candidates and can only attract bonus marks. In Appendix 1 you will find a collection of the more famous of these eponyms. The Examiners would want you to know the description of the eponym and the country of origin and occupation of the person it was called after (most, but not all, were obstetricians and gynaecologists).

Sample oral assessment stations

Station 1

This is a preparatory station. You are provided here with the following patient's information leaflet. Please read it in preparation for the next station where you will be asked to critically appraise it.

Patient's Information Leaflet
Laparoscopic Sterilization

You will be having a laparoscopic sterilization operation. This is usually done as a day-case, in which you are admitted, have the operation and go home on the same day. The operation will be performed under general anaesthesia and involves inserting a scope through a small (1 cm) cut at the umbilicus to have a look at the fallopian tubes, where the egg and sperm normally meet. By blocking these tubes the sperm will be prevented from meeting the egg and you will not be able to get pregnant. The tubes are blocked by applying special clips or rings to them using an instrument inserted through another small cut in the abdomen.

The operation is irreversible; once it is done it can not be undone. However, there is a chance that it might fail and some women will get pregnant after having the operation. This happens once in every 200 cases (5 per 1000). If you become pregnant after sterilization, there is a high chance that this pregnancy could be in the tube (ectopic pregnancy). This is a serious condition that can be life-threatening and usually requires an operation to sort it out. Also, in some women the operation makes the period heavier and slightly more frequent.

Station 2

In this station you will critically appraise the leaflet you were given in the previous station, and discuss it with the Examiner.

Examiners' Instructions

There are a number of deficiencies and inaccuracies in the information, and marks should be awarded if the candidate detects them as follows:

- No mention of possible operative complications (injuries, bleeding, the need for laparotomy)   **2 Marks**

- The leaflet states the operation is irreversible. This is not strictly correct (reversal success rate ~ 60%). Rather it should be 'considered' irreversible as irreversibility is unpredictable. The woman may know someone who has had a sterilization successfully reversed, thus undermining her confidence in the accuracy of the leaflet.   **2 Marks**

- It states that the operation causes the period to become heavier. This was suggested by earlier studies but was found, later on, to be incorrect.   **2 Marks**

- The candidate should be aware of the recent controversy about the long-term (10-year) failure rate for some methods (up to 35 per 1000). This has not been yet assessed for Filshie clip.   **2 Marks**

- Presentation and Examiner's discretion.   **2 Marks**

                                   Total Mark   10

Station 3

A 25-year-old woman is requesting emergency contraception. You are required to discuss with the Examiner how you would counsel this patient and the different options you are going to offer her.

Examiners' Instructions
The marks should be awarded as follows:

- Good history-taking of timing of all instances of unprotected intercourse in current cycle   **1 Mark**

- Past medical history (contraindications).   **1 Mark**

- Yuzpe method.   **2 Marks**

- IUCD.   **2 Marks**

- Progestogen-only method, and knowledge of the recent data indicating that it is more successful than the combined (Yuzpe) method.   **2 Marks**

- Presentation and Examiner's discretion.   **2 Marks**

                                   Total Mark   10

Station 4

This 35-year-old patient had a routine smear which showed moderate dyskaryosis. She has been referred by her GP to the gynaecology clinic where you are seeing her now. How would you deal with this patient?

Examiners Instructions

In this station the candidate explains to the role-player while being observed by the Examiners.

The role-player should ask the candidate the following questions:

Is this cancer?

What happens now?

Will I have to have a hysterectomy?

Both the Examiner and the role-player assess the candidate as follows

For the Examiner

- Introduction.   **1 Mark**

- Put patient at ease.   **1 Mark**

- Listen attentively.   **1 Mark**

- Explain the condition.   **1 Mark**

- Avoidance of medical jargon.   **1 Mark**

- Verbal and non-verbal clues followed.   **1 Mark**

- Intended action explained.   **1 Mark**

- Appropriate eye contact.   **1 Mark**

For the role-payer

- Confidence in candidate.   **1 Mark**

- I would like to see this doctor again.   **1 Mark**

                                               Total Mark   10

Station 5

Describe why and how to do a laparoscopic ovarian drilling.

Examiners' Instructions

The marks should be awarded as follows. If the candidate does not provide these answers unprompted, the Examiners should ask the questions:

- Indication: CC resistant PCOS.   **1 Mark**

- Basic laparoscopic technique.   **3 Marks**

- Techniques of ovarian drilling.   **1 Mark**

- Expected results.   **2 Marks**
- Alternative: gonadotrophin ovulation induction   **1 Mark**
- Advantages of ovarian drilling: one-step treatment and
  mono ovulation.   **2 Marks**

  Total Mark   **10**

Station 6

A 31-year-old patient with a 1-year history of primary infertility was fully investigated, and only mild endometriosis was detected. Her partner had a normal seminal fluid analysis. How would you proceed?

Examiners Instructions

- The marks should be awarded as follows:
- Mild endometriosis reduces fertility.   **1 Mark**
- Ablation of endometriotic lesions (diathermy/laser) effective.   **2 Marks**
- Danazol not effective.   **1 Mark**
- GnRH agonists not effective.   **1 Mark**
- High chance of spontaneous pregnancy.   **2 Marks**
- Superovulation/IUI.   **1 Mark**
- Presentation and Examiner's discretion.   **2 Marks**

  Total Mark   **10**

Station 7

This is a preparatory station. You are asked to design an audit protocol to find out if postnatal patients at high risk of thromboembolic complications are receiving subcutaneous prophylactic heparin in your hospital. You will be asked in the next station to explain your protocol to the Examiner who will discuss it with you.

Station 8

In this station you will present your audit protocol from the previous station, and discuss it with the Examiner.

Examiners Instructions

The marks should be awarded as follows:

- Establishing a gold standard to measure practice against
  (e.g. for all CS). **2 Marks**

- Collecting data on actual practice. **2 Marks**

- Analysing these data and comparing them to the gold
  standard. **2 Marks**

- Presenting the results with suggestions on how to improve
  practice. **2 Marks**

- Implementing these suggestions and re-auditing after a
  reasonable period. **2 Marks**

  Total Mark 10

Station 9

The candidate is given a pair of Kielland's forceps and a pair of Simpson's forceps.

Examiners' Instructions

The questions asked and marks awarded should be as follows:

- What are these called? **2 Marks**

- Conditions to be fulfilled before applying forceps. **2 Marks**

- Primigravida at term, uncomplicated pregnancy. Pushing
  in the second stage for 2 hours. Fetal head 1/5th
  abdominally. +1 vaginally. DOA. What is next?
  Answers to be complete must include trial in theatre
  (or CS). **4 Marks**

- Presentation and Examiner's discretion. **2 Marks**

  Total Mark 10

Station 10

This 25-year-old pregnant woman at 17 weeks' gestation had a high maternal serum AFP. You are seeing her in the antenatal clinic to explain the results.

Examiners' Instructions

In this station the candidate explains to the role-player while being observed by the Examiners.

The role-player should ask the candidate the following questions:
Is the baby abnormal?
Can you do a test to guarantee that all will be well?
Will I loose the baby?

Both the Examiner and the role-player assess the candidate as follows:
For the Examiner

- Introduction.   **1 Mark**

- Put patient at ease.   **1 Mark**

- Listen attentively.   **1 Mark**

- Explain the condition.   **1 Mark**

- Avoidance of medical jargon.   **1 Mark**

- Verbal and non-verbal clues followed.   **1 Mark**

- Intended action explained.   **1 Mark**

- Appropriate eye contact.   **1 Mark**

For the role-player

- Confidence in candidate.   **1 Mark**

- I would like to see this doctor again.   **1 Mark**

                                      Total Mark   10

Station 11

A 33-year-old known epileptic and her husband have come to see you for counselling. She is currently taking sodium valproate (Epilim) which was found to be the only drug to control her fits effectively. They would like to start a family.

Examiners' Instructions

The following questions should be asked, and the marks awarded as follows:

- What pre-pregnancy advice would you offer her?
  Continue with the drug.   **1 Mark**
  Take folic acid.   **1 Mark**

- What is the main complication of epilim on the fetus?
  NTD. **2 Marks**

- So what needs to be done during pregnancy?
  Detailed USS. **1 Mark**

- What may happen to her epilepsy during pregnancy?
  Increased drug requirements. **1 Mark**

- Why?
  N+V, increased blood volume, increased binding globulins. **3 Marks**

- Presentation and Examiner's discretion. **1 Mark**

  Total Mark 10

Station 12

A 33-year-old woman has presented to the casualty department with mild lower abdominal pain and slight vaginal spotting. She was unsure of the date of her last menstrual period. Examination was unremarkable and a urine pregnancy test was positive. A transvaginal scan showed a thickened endometrium and no intrauterine sac. What is your management?

Examiners' Instructions
Within the answer, the Examiner should explore the candidate's knowledge about the following:

- Serum beta-hCG and the concept of the discriminatory zone. **2 Marks**

- Diagnostic laparoscopy. **2 Marks**

- Laparoscopic treatment versus laparotomy. **2 Marks**

- Methotrexate treatment. **1 Mark**

- Overall answer and Examiner's discretion. **3 Marks**

  Total Mark 10

KEY POINTS

- The oral assessment examination consists of a circuit containing 12 stations, with 15 minutes allocated to each. Ten of these stations are 'active' and have an Examiner present, and two stations are 'preparatory' for the following station.

- There are no real patients in the examination, but some stations have role-players depicting a particular clinical scenario.

- Your clinical competence, factual knowledge, analytical thinking, professional communication skills and ability to formulate management plans will be assessed during the examination.

- Effective communication, attention to detail and a clinical approach are the essential tools of success in the examination.

- Different types of questions may be asked, each requiring different approaches in the answer.

- Read the instructions, listen to the Examiner and role-player, understand the question and think before you answer.

- If in difficulty, reflect on your clinical practice and think how you will manage a similar problem in the hospital.

- Do not argue with the Examiners.

14

Literature Appraisal for the MRCOG Examination

With special contribution from Mr. Khalid Khan, MRCOG.

Introduction

Literature appraisal is a skill doctors cannot live without. Gone are the days when all what you needed to know for your professional life was present in textbooks. Advances in medicine are making most textbooks out of date by the time they are published. In order to keep your practice up-to-date you have to use the literature. This comes in many shapes and forms; printed, electronic, internet, original papers, meta-analysis, reviews, case reports, guidelines, information leaflets, etc. It also comes with variable degrees of quality. It is essential that you are able to appraise the different types of literature and assess their quality in order to find out if you should, or should not, change your practice based upon them. Recognizing the importance of this issue, the RCOG has dedicated at least one station of the Oral Assessment Examination in the Part 2 MRCOG to literature appraisal, as we have discussed in the previous chapter. In this chapter we describe how to critically appraise the literature you may be presented with at the MRCOG examination.

Literature appraisal

A paradigm shift in clinical practice is integrating individual clinical expertise with published evidence in the literature. This paradigm is called evidence-based medicine and it enhances the quality of patient management enabling

Table 2: Levels of evidence.

Level	Type of evidence
I	Evidence obtained from at least one randomized controlled trial or from meta-analysis of randomized controlled trials
II	Evidence obtained from at least one well-designed controlled study without randomization
III	Evidence obtained from well-designed non-experimental descriptive studies, such as comparative studies, correlation studies and case control studies
IV	Evidence obtained from expert committee reports or opinions and/or clinical experience of respected authorites

achievement of the best possible clinical outcome. The MRCOG exam will formally test you in appraisal of the published literature. You will probably be given a paper of one to two pages to read at a preparatory station followed by questions and discussion with the Examiner at the next station. This makes it more likely that the reading material will be a short report, either a case report, summary of a clinical practice guideline or a patient information leaflet. Before we move on to the specifics of appraising these publication types, let us look at some general principles of literature evaluation which will come in handy in critically looking at any articles you are faced with. You should first be aware that publications in the medical literature are grouped according to their quality known as the levels of evidence, as shown in Table 2. The levels are a general guide to determining how rigorous and credible the publication might be. The published literature often mixes the few rigorous studies (levels I and II) with the many not so rigorous studies (levels Ill and IV). It will be your job as the candidate to determine whether the information presented to you is based on rigorous evidence or not.

Appraisal of case reports

You will have noticed from Table 2 that case reports are regarded as the lowest level of evidence. This is because their methods do not permit discrimination of the scientifically valid from the interesting only publications. However, case reports and anecdotal information exert a powerful influence on clinical behaviour. Therefore all major journals devote some space to publishing case reports. They are intended to implant clinically-useful reminders in clinicians' heads. You should view case reports as communications between clinicians and ask yourself the following questions:

- What was the cause of the patient's illness?

- Were all available therapeutic options considered?

- What would you have done and would you do things differently in a similar case in the future?

Most case reports would not be rarities; rather they would be common problems with unusual presentation or difficult management. In addressing the above questions you should bring to bear in your mind the knowledge of the full range of diagnostic work-up for a clinical presentation. This will help determine if the patient's illness was diagnosed correctly in timely manner. Following a diagnosis you need to determine if all therapeutic options were considered and if the most appropriate one was chosen given the individual patient's circumstances. Finally, you need to consider if the knowledge of this case helps you manage similar patients in the future more effectively.

Appraisal of clinical practice guidelines

The purpose of clinical guidelines is to improve the effectiveness and efficiency of clinical care through the identification of good clinical practice and desired clinical outcomes. Clinical practice guidelines are systemetically-developed statements to assist practitioner and patient in decisions about appropriate health care for specific clinical circumstances. Generally each one of the statements is graded for its value according to the level of evidence that lies behind the recommendation. And just to make things difficult for all of us the grades of recommendations are lettered differently to the levels of evidence (Table 3). One could appraise guidelines asking three basic questions about them:

- What are the recommendations?

- Are they valid?

- Will they help in patient care?

Practice guidelines represent an attempt to distil a large body of medical knowledge into a convenient, readily usable format. They gather, appraise

Table 3: Grading of recommendations.

Grade	Recommendation
A	(Evidence level I) Requires at least one randomized controlled trial as part of the body of literature of overall good quality and consistency addressing the specific recommendation
B	(Evidence levels II, III) Requires availability of well-conducted clinical studies but not randomized clinical trials on the topic of recommendation
C	(Evidence level IV) Requires evidence from expert committee reports or opinions and/or clinical experience of respected authorites. Indicates absence of directly applicable studies of good quality

and combine evidence in attempting to address all issues relevant to a clinical decision. The value of clinical guidelines rests on ensuring validity – the available evidence is correctly synthesized and weighted within a guideline so that, when followed, the guideline leads to improvements in health. Guidelines are about clinical decision-making and decisions involve choices and consequences. You need to check if all the reasonable practice options and their outcomes have been considered in the guideline you are appraising.

Many guidelines are developed by expert groups without formal literature reviews. This approach relies heavily upon the group's knowledge of the literature and its members' experience of routine clinical practice. However, clinicians' knowledge of the literature is often incomplete and their clinical experience may be biased, causing them to overestimate or underestimate effectiveness of treatments. Systematic literature reviews overcome these problems by using an explicit search strategy and inclusion criteria to identify evidence. You should see if the guideline developers used an explicit and sensible process to identify, select and summarize evidence. They should by able to account for important recent developments. In the absence of information about how the evidence was selected and evaluated, you cannot appraise the guideline. As many guidelines are produced without formal publication in journals, they are usually not externally peer-reviewed. In order for the guideline to be valid, you should look for evidence that the guideline was subjected to an internal peer review process. The reviewers should have judged the conclusions reasonable and applicable in practice.

Once you are satisfied that the guideline was developed using rigorous methodology, your confidence in its clinical usefulness should vary according to the strength of the evidence on which it is based. The guideline should provide graded recommendations on key issues based on levels of evidence (Table 3) and best practice for the delivery of patient-centred care. The extent to which guidelines will help in patient care should depend on whether the recommendations are applicable to your patients. Generally, the guidelines should be initially viewed for use as a starting point and then developed through local discussion (at clinical directorate, ward, general practice, or other appropriate levels) and agreed locally.

Appraisal of patient information leaflets

Just as scientific literature is being used to support medical decision-making, patients' decision-making is increasingly being supported by written information about their condition and its treatment. Patients have the right to be given factual, supportable, understandable and appropriate information, to be provided in such a way as to allow them to decide whether they wish to receive therapy. Thus patient information leaflets are the currency of therapeutic dialogue. In appraising the leaflets you should ask yourself the following questions:

- Is the leaflet up-to-date?

- Is the information in the leaflet appropriate and reliable?

- Is it presented in a usable way?

With scientific advancement, medical knowledge is growing at a fast pace. Patient information leaflets should keep pace with these developments. Without an attempt to keep current the information in patient leaflets is bound to become outdated very soon. The leaflets should clearly specify the date of the last revisions in the information. For each clinical situation, what information is essential, desirable and optional, depends very much on the purpose of the leaflet. You should consider if the leaflet is meant to provide information about a health state or it is describing an operation the patient is being offered. The appropriateness of the information included will vary in the two situations. For the leaflets to be reliable, they should contain information consistent with the standards of health care according to current best evidence. Here you will have to consider if any new developments have been missed or if any undesirable options are included. Finally, you should consider if the material is presented to the level of communication of the abilities and needs of the patients, i.e. is written in lay-person's terms. If the patients have difficulty understanding, is there an additional source or contact included to which patients might turn to for help or explanation?

Appendix 1

Eponyms – Who's Who in Obstetrics and Gynaecology

Introduction

Love them or hate them, eponyms are here to stay. Life would never be the same again if you had to ask for 'long shanked rotational forceps with minimal pelvic curve' instead of 'Kielland forceps' or for a self-retaining trans-urethral urinary catheter' instead of a 'Foley's catheter'. Eponyms make you recognize the contributions of your predecessors and help to put a human touch and a breath of life into the stone-cold medical sciences. If all this does not convince you, then the following should: they are common questions in the examination! Your Examiners have spent most of their lives practising obstetrics and gynaecology and they sincerely hope that their contributions, and those of others before them, would not be forgotten.

By this stage of your medical training, you must have been through so many examinations, and have come to realize that they are all about making good impressions. If asked 'Who was Kielland?' you will not fail for not knowing the answer, but surely it will be far better if you did. At least it will save you from saying that most dreaded and demoralizing answer in any examination: 'I don't know'. We agree that most candidates would probably not know the answer, but wouldn't it be more impressive if you were one of the few who did?

In this chapter we have listed (alphabetically) the more common eponyms in the field of obstetrics and gynaecology. The name of the person is printed in **bold**, followed by their year of birth (and death) if known. This is mainly done to distinguish the contemporaries. Following that, there is a short biographical note. The name of the eponym is printed in *italic* followed by a brief description. We have included more names than we think is necessary for the MRCOG, as we believe this might be useful for you in your future career.

- **ANDREWS, Henry** (1871–1942). Consultant Obstetrician and Gynaecologist at the London Hospital.
  Brandt-Andrews Manoeuvre: Delivery of the placenta by controlled cord traction and abdominal pressure.

- **APGAR, Virginia** (1909–1974). American anaesthetist.
  Apgar Score: Scoring system for neonatal assessment at birth (described 1953).

- **ARIAS–STELLA, Javier** (born 1920). Lima pathologist.
  Arias-Stella's Phenomenon: Atypical changes in the cell nuclei of the endometrium due to increased gonadotrophin stimulation. Before the description by Arias-Stella (in 1954) they were confused with carcinoma cells.

- **ARNOLD, Julius** (1835–1915). Professor of Pathological Anatomy, Heidelberg.
  Arnold–Chiari Malformation: Hind-brain anomaly in which the cerebellar tonsils and medulla are malformed and herniate through the foramen magnum causing progressive obstructive hydrocephalus (described 1894).

- **ASHERMAN, Joseph.** Tel-Aviv gynaecologist.
  Asherman Syndrome: Intrauterine synechiae.

- **AYRE, James Ernest** (1910–1974). Director, Papanicolaou Cancer Research Institute, Miami, Florida.
  Ayre's Spatula: Special spatula for collecting cervical smears.

- **BANDL, Ludwig** (1842–1892). Vienna gynaecologist.
  Bandl's Ring: Pathological retraction ring between the lower and the upper uterine segments in cases of obstructed labour. A sign of impending uterine rupture.

- **BARNES, Robert** (1817–1907). President of the Obstetric Society of London.
  Neville–Barnes Forceps: Long, curved obstetric forceps.

- **BARR, Murray** (born 1908). Head of the Department of Anatomy, University of Western Ontario.
  Barr Body: Sex chromatin body (described 1949).

- **BARTHOLIN, Caspar** (1655–1738). Professor of Anatomy, Medicine and Physics at the University of Copenhagen.
  Bartholin's Gland: Greater vestibular glands (described 1677).

- **BEHCET, Halushi** (1889–1948). Turkish dermatologist.
  Behcet's Syndrome: Recurrent progressive disease of unknown cause affecting many organs: painful labial (scrotal) and oral ulcerations which heal by scarring, arthritis, keratitis, iritis, meningioencephalitis, Parkinsonism, dementia and thrombophlebitis (described 1937).

- **BONNEY, William Francis Victor** (1872–1953). Gynaecologist at the Middlesex Hospital, the Royal Masonic Hospital, the Chelsea Hospital for Women and the Postgraduate Medical School, London. His contributions to gynaecological surgery were mainly in the fields of radical pelvic surgery and conservative surgery for fibroids. It was a sad irony that, before he pioneered myomectomy, his wife had a sub-total hysterectomy for a single submucous fibroid.
  Bonney's Gynaecological Surgery: Famous textbook (first edition 1911).
  Bonney's Blue: Skin-marking ink.
  Bonney's Test: Elevation of bladder neck during vaginal examination reduces the urine loss in stress incontinence.
  Bonney's Gynaecological Scissors.
  Bonney's Myomectomy Clamps: Special clamps used to compress the uterine arteries at the base of the broad ligament during myomectomy operation.
  Bonney's Hood Myomectomy: Myomectomy using anterior hood-type incision to prevent the formation of adhesions to the bowels.

- **BOWEN, John Templeton** (1857–1941). Professor of Dermatology, Harvard University, Boston.
  Bowen's Disease (of the vulva): Vulval intra-epithelial neoplasia (described 1912).

- **BRANDT, Thure** (1819–1895). Stockholm Obstetrician and Gynaecologist.
  Brandt–Andrews Manoeuvre: see Andrews.

- **BRAXTON-HICKS, John** (1825–1897). Obstetrician and Gynaecologist to Guy's Hospital, London. He also described bipolar (combined external and internal) version in 1860.
  Braxton-Hicks Contractions: Intermittent uterine contractions prior to the onset of labour (described 1871).

- **CAMPER, Pieter** (1722–1789). Professor of Medicine, Amsterdam.
  Camper's Fascia: Superficial layer of the superficial fascia of the abdominal wall.

- **von CHIARI, Hans** (1851–1916). Professor of Pathological Anatomy at Strasbourg.
  Arnold–Chiari Malformation: see Arnold.

- **CLOQUET, Jules Gemain** (1790–1883). Professor of Anatomy and Surgery in Paris, Surgeon to Napoleon III and President of the French Academy of Medicine.
  Lymph Gland of Cloquet: Lymphatic gland at the apex of the femoral canal (described 1817).

- **COOMBS, Robin** (born 1921). Professor of Biology and Head of Immunology Division, University of Cambridge.
  Coombs' Test: Antiglobulin test to detect red cells antibodies.

- **COOPER, Astley** (1768–1841). Surgeon to St Thomas's and Guy's Hospitals in 1800. Later he became Professor at Surgeons' Hall and President of the Royal Medical and Chirurgical Society, and of the Royal College of Surgeons.
  Cooper' Fascia: Covering of the spermatic cord (described 1804).
  Cooper's Ligaments: Skin attachments of the breast (described 1840).

- **COUVELAIRE, Alexandre** (1873–1948). Paris obstetrician.
  Couvelaire Uterus (uterine apoplexy): Extravasation of blood (resulting from placental abruption) into the uterine wall musculature (described 1911).

- **COWPER, William** (1666–1709). London surgeon.
  Cowper's Glands: Bulbo-urethral glands (described 1700).

- **CREDE, Karl Sigmund** (1819–1892). Berlin-born obstetrician who became the Professor of Obstetrics at Leipzig. He introduced the use of silver nitrate eye-drops to prevent ophthalmia neonatorum (1884).
  Crede's Manoeuvre: External uterine pressure to expel the placenta (described 1860).

- **CULLEN, Thomas Stephen** (1868–1953). Professor of Gynaecology at Johns Hopkins University, Baltimore.
  Cullen's Sign: Bluish discolouration around the umbilicus in pancreatitis and intra-abdominal haemorrhage, originally described in a case of ruptured ectopic pregnancy (1919).

- **DÖDERLEIN, Albert Siegmund Gustav** (1860–1941). Professor of Gynaecology at Johns Hopkins University, Baltimore.
  Döderlein Bacillus: Gram-positive micro-organism found in the vagina and responsible for its normal acidity.

- **DONOVAN, Charles** (1863–1951). Irish-trained Professor of Physiology at Madras College, India.
  Donovan Bodies: Gram-negative rods of *Donovania granulomatis*, found in the cytoplasm of mononuclear cells in cases of granuloma venereum (described 1905).

- **DOPPLER, Christian Johann** (1803–1853). Austrian physicist and mathematician.
  Doppler Effect: Relationship between observed frequency of sound or light waves to the relative movement of the source and observer (described 1842).

- **DOUGLAS, James** (1675–1742). London anatomist and 'man-midwife', who became Physician to Queen Caroline, the wife of George II.
  Pouch of Douglas: Recto-uterine peritoneal pouch (described 1730).
  Semicircular Fold of Douglas: Lower margin of the posterior rectus sheath, situated an inch below the level of the umbilicus (described 1730).

- **DOWN, John Langdon Haydon** (1828–1896). Assistant Physician at the London Hospital Medical College. He was also the Medical Superintendent at Earlswood Asylum for Idiots, Redhill, and founded Normansfield Mental Hospital.
  Down's Syndrome: Classically trisomy 21, but 5% of cases are due to translocation (described 1866).

- **DUCHENNE, Guillaume Benjamin** (1806–1875). Paris neurologist.
  Erb–Duchenne Palsy: Brachial plexus palsy involving the upper roots (C5,6,7), and causing weakness of the shoulder muscles, biceps, brachioradialis and the supinators of the forearm (waiter's tip position). Classically a birth injury resulting from excessive traction on the fetal head (described 1855 by Duchenne and 1874 by Erb).

- **ERB, Wilhelm** (1840–1921). Professor of Medicine at Leipzig and Heidelberg.
  Erb–Duchenne Palsy: see Duchenne.

- **FALLOPIO, Gabriele** (1523–1563). Professor of Surgery, Anatomy and Botany at Padua, Italy.
  Fallopian Tubes: Oviducts (described 1561).

- **FOLEY, Frederic Eugene Basil** (1891–1966). Urologist, Miller and Ancker Hospitals, St Paul, Minnesota.
  Foley's Catheter: Self-retaining urinary catheter.

- **FREI, Wilhelm Siegmund** (1885–1943). Professor of Dermatology at the State Hospital, Spandau, Berlin.
  Frei Test: Intradermal test for lymphogranuloma venereum (described 1925).

- **GAERTNER, Hermann** (1785–1827). Anatomist and surgeon in the Norwegian Army.
  Gaertner's Duct: Remnant of the lower end of the Wolffian duct which can lead to a cystic swelling in the vaginal wall.

- **de GRAAF, Regnier** (1641–1673). He was born in Holland and worked as an Anatomist and Physician in France.
  Graafian Follicle: Mature ovarian follicle (described 1672).

- **GREEN-ARMYTAGE, Vivian Bartley** (1882–1961). Professor of Obstetrics and Gynaecology in Calcutta and later Obstetrician and Gynaecologist at the West London Hospital and the British Postgraduate Hospital.
  Green-Armytage Forceps: Forceps used for holding the edges of the uterine incision at Caesarean section.

- **HEGAR, Alfred** (1830–1914). Professor of Obstetrics and Gynaecology in Freiburg.
  Hegar's Dilator: Metal graded cervical dilators.

- **HODGE, Hugh** (1796–1873). Philadelphia obstetrician and gynaecologist.
  Smith–Hodge Pessary: Vaginal pessary for correction of uterine retroversion (described 1866).

- **HUHNER, Max** (1873–1974). New York urologist.
  Sims–Huhner Test: Post/coital test.

- **KALLAMAN, Frank** (1897–1945). New York psychiatrist.
  Kallaman's Syndrome: Olfacto-genital syndrome.

- **KIELLAND, Christian** (1871–1941). Norwegian obstetrician and gynaecologist.
  Kielland Forceps: (described 1915).

- **KLINEFELTER, Harry** (born 1912). Associate Professor of Medicine, Johns Hopkins Medical School, Baltimore.
  Klinefelter's Syndrome: Male hypergonadotrophic hypogonadism with sex chromosome aneuploidy (47XXY) (described 1942).

- **KLUMPKE, Augusta** (1859–1927). Paris neurologist.
Klumpke's Paralysis: Brachial plexus palsy involving the lower roots (C8,T1), and causing weakness of the small muscles of the forearm and hand. Classically a birth injury resulting from excessive traction on the fetal head (described 1885).

- **KRUKENBERG, Friedrich** (1871–1946). Pathologist and Professor of Ophthalmology, Halle.
Krukenberg Tumour: Metastatic, usually bilateral, ovarian carcinoma with primary malignancy usually located in the gastrointestinal tract (described 1896).

- **von LANGER, Carl** (1819–1887). Professor of Zoology, Budapest.
Langer's Lines: Tension lines in the skin due to the arrangement of the dermis collagen fibres (described 1861).

- **LEVENTHAL, Michael** (1901–1971). American obstetrician and gynaecologist.
Stein–Leventhal Syndrome: Polycystic ovarian disease (described 1935).

- **von LEYDIG, Franz** (1821–1908). Professor of Histology, Wurzburg.
Leydig Cells: Interstitial cells of the testis (described 1850).

- **LØVSET, Jørgen** (1631-1691). Norwegian obstetrician.
Løvset's Manoeuvre: Rotation of the fetal trunk to assist delivery of the arms in breech delivery.

- **MACKENRODT, Alwin** (1859–1925). Professor of Gynaecology, Berlin.
Mackenrodt's Ligament: Transverse cervical ligament (described 1895).

- **MEIGS, Joseph** (1892–1963). Professor of Gynaecology at Harvard University.
Meigs' Syndrome: Ovarian fibroma, ascites and (usually right-sided) pleural effusion (described 1937).

- **MENDEL, Gregor** (1822–1884). Austrian monk and the founder of modern genetics.
Mendel's Law: Independent assortment and segregation of inherited factors (described 1865).

- **MENDELSON, Curtis**. Contemporary American obstetrician and gynaecologist, New York Hospital.
Mendelson's Syndrome: Chemical pneumonitis resulting from aspiration of

acidic gastric contents during general anaesthesia due to abolition of laryngeal reflex (described 1945).

- **MÜLLER, Johannes** (1801–1858). Professor of Anatomy and Physiology, Berlin.
  Müllerian Duct: Paramesonephric duct (described 1825).

- **NABOTH, Martin** (1675–1721). Professor of Medicine, Leipzig.
  Nabothian Follicles: Retention cysts of the cervical mucous glands (described 1707).

- **NAEGELE, Franz** (1777–1851). Heidelberg obstetrician.
  Naegele's Rule: Formula for calculating the expected date of delivery from the first day of the last menstrual period (+7 days, +9 months).

- **NEISSER, Albert** (1855–1916). Director of Dermatological Institute, Breslau.
  Neisseria gonorrhoea: Gram-negative diplococci.

- **NEVILLE, William** (died 1904). Obstetrician, Rotunda Hospital, Dublin.
  Neville–Barnes Forceps: Long curved obstetric forceps (Neville added the axis-traction piece to Barnes's original forceps).

- **PAGET, Sir James** (1814–1899). Surgeon at St Bartholomew Hospital and President of the Royal College of Surgeons, London.
  Paget's Disease: of the vulva/ penis/ breast/ bone.

- **PAPANICOLAOU, George** (1884–1962). Professor of Anatomy, Cornell University, New York.
  Papanicolaou Smear: Cervical smear (described 1933).

- **PATAU, Klaus**. American paediatrician.
  Patau's Syndrome: Trisomy 13.

- **PFANNENSTIEL, Hermann** (1862–1909). Breslau gynaecologist.
  Pfannenstiel's Incision: Suprapubic transverse abdominal incision cutting the skin, subcutaneous tissue and fascia transversely (described 1900).

- **PINARD, Adolphe** (1844–1934). Paris obstetrician.
  Pinard's Stethoscope.

- **POUPART, Francois** (1661–1709). Paris surgeon.
  Poupart's Ligament: Inguinal ligament (described 1705).

- **RUBIN, Isidor Clinton** (1883–1958). Gynaecologist at Mount Sinai Hospital and Beth Israel Hospital, New York.
  Rubin's Test: Tubal patency test.

- **SCARPA, Antonio** (1747–1832). Italian anatomist and surgeon.
  Scarpa's Fascia: Deep layer of the superficial fascia of the abdominal wall (described 1809).
  Scarpa's Triangle: Femoral triangle.

- **SCHAUTA, Friedrich** (1849–1919). Vienna gynaecologist.
  Schauta's Operation: Radical vaginal hysterectomy.

- **SCHILLER, Walter** (1887–1960). Vienna gynaecologist and pathologist.
  Schiller's Test: Painting the cervix with 3–5% Lugol's iodine to demarcate abnormal epithelium.

- **SERTOLI, Enrico** (1842–1910). Professor of Physiology, Milan.
  Sertoli Cells: Cells of the seminiferous tubules (described 1865).

- **SHEEHAN, Harold** (born 1900). Professor of Pathology, Liverpool University.
  Sheehan's Syndrome: Postpartum hypopituitarism, due to necrosis usually secondary to severe postpartum haemorrhage.

- **SIMPSON, James Young** (1811–1870). Professor of Obstetrics, Edinburgh.
  Simpson's Forceps: Long, curved obstetric forceps (described 1848).

- **SIMS, Harry**. Boston gynaecologist.
  Sims–Huhner Test: see Huhner.

- **SIMS, James Marion** (1813–1883). American gynaecologist and pioneer of vesico-vaginal fistula repair.
  Sims' Speculum: Vaginal speculum (Sims originally used a bent spoon in 1852).
  Sims' Position.

- **SKENE, Alexander** (1838–1900). Originally from Aberdeen. Professor of Gynaecology at Long Island College Hospital, New York.
  Skene's Ducts: Paraurethral glands in the female (described 1880).

- **STEIN, Irving** (born 1887). Chicago gynaecologist.
  Stein–Leventhal Syndrome: see Leventhal.

- **TRENDELENBURG, Friedrich** (1844–1924). Professor of Surgery, Bonn.
  Trendelenburg Position: Head-down operating position (described 1890).

- **TURNER, Henry** (born 1892). Professor of Medicine, Oklahoma University, USA.
  Turner's Syndrome: Ovarian dysgenesis, 45XO.

- **WASSERMANN, August** (1866–1925). Director of the Department of Therapeutic and Serum Research, University of Berlin.
  Wassermann Reaction: Complement fixation test for the diagnosis of syphilis (described 1906).

- **WERTHEIM, Ernst** (1864–1920). Vienna gynaecologist.
  Wertheim's Operation: Radical hysterectomy (described 1900).

- **WOLFF, Kaspar** (1733–1794). Professor of Anatomy and Physiology at St Petersburg.
  Wolffian Duct: Mesonephric duct (described 1759).

Appendix 2

A Guide to MRCOG Courses

Introduction

'Should I go to a course before the examination?' This question is commonly asked by many prospective Part 1 and Part 2 examination candidates. The answer must be 'yes'. This does not mean that you are unlikely to pass unless you attend a course; many candidates do. It simply means that you will, on balance, increase your chances of success if you attend a course. The term 'course' here is used in its narrow context, which means MRCOG-orientated courses. This does not include other educational courses which are not specifically exam-orientated. These are very useful, but are beyond the scope of this discussion.

The pass rate in both parts of the MRCOG is between 30 and 40%, which means that, on average, 6 out of 10 candidates will fail. Every help, therefore, is needed. The fact that you are reading this book indicates that you have already recognized this basic concept. Some would argue that good candidates do not need such help as attending courses. The compelling counter argument, however, is that those 'good' candidates are only known in retrospect, after they have passed the examination. Moreover, every candidate can become a 'good' candidate with the appropriate preparation. Courses form a part of this preparation.

Here we have presented a list of some of the courses for the Part 1 and Part 2 examinations. For each course, we have listed the venue, dates, duration, components and address for correspondence.

Courses for the Part 1 MRCOG

- **Royal College of Obstetricians & Gynaecologists MRCOG Part 1 Revision Course**

Venue:	RCOG, London.
Dates & Duration:	January / July (1 week).
Components:	Lectures and MCQ practice.
Correspondence address:	Postgraduate Education Department, RCOG, 27 Sussex Place, Regent's Park, London NW1 4RG, UK Tel: 0171–772 6200.

- **University of Nottingham MRCOG Part 1 Course**

Venue:	Medical School, University of Nottingham.
Dates & Duration:	January / July (2 weeks).
Components:	Lectures and MCQ practice.
Correspondence address:	Postgraduate Course Co-ordinator, Department of Obstetrics & Gynaecology, University Hospital, Queen's Medical Centre, Nottingham NG7 2UH, UK Tel: 0115–970 9451.

- **Queen Charlotte's Hospital Course in Basic Medical Sciences for MRCOG Part 1**

Venue:	Institute of Obstetrics & Gynaecology, Queen Charlotte's & Chelsea Hospital, London.
Dates & Duration:	June / December (2 weeks).
Components:	Lectures and MCQ practice.
Correspondence address:	Courses Secretary, Institute of Obstetrics & Gynaecology, Queen Charlotte's & Chelsea Hospital, Goldhawk Road, London W6 OXG, UK Tel: 0181–383 3902.

● Newcastle MRCOG Part 1 Course

Venue:	Royal Victoria Infirmary, Newcastle upon Tyne.
Dates & Duration:	January/ July (2 weeks).
Components:	Lectures and MCQ practice.
Correspondence address:	The Registrar, Regional Postgraduate Institute of Medicine & Dentistry, The University, 11 Framlington Place, Newcastle upon Tyne NE2 4AB, UK Tel: 0191–222 6762.

● Edinburgh Postgraduate Board MRCOG Part 1 Course

Venue:	Lister Postgraduate Institute, Edinburgh.
Dates & Duration:	January (2 weeks).
Components:	Lectures and MCQ practice.
Correspondence address:	The Postgraduate Dean, Edinburgh Postgraduate Board for Medicine, Pfizer Foundation, 11 Hill Square, Edinburgh EH8 9DR, UK Tel: 0131–650 2609.

● University of Keele MRCOG Part 1 Course

Venue:	North Staffordshire Hospital Centre, Stoke-on-Trent.
Dates & Duration:	November (2 weeks).
Components:	Lectures and MCQ practice.
Correspondence address:	Part 1 MRCOG Course Secretary, School of Postgraduate Medicine & Biological Sciences, Thornburrow Drive, Hartshill, Stoke-on-Trent ST4 7QB, UK Tel: 01782–716 998.

- **Liverpool MRCOG Part 1 Course**

Venue:	Mill Road Maternity Hospital, Liverpool.
Dates & Duration:	November–February (weekly half-day release)
Components:	Lectures.
Correspondence address:	MRCOG Course Secretary, Postgraduate Course Co-ordinator's Office, Mill Road Maternity Hospital, Liverpool L6 2AH, UK Tel: 0151–260 8787 Ext. 2748.

- **University Examination Postal Institution MRCOG Part 1 Correspondence Course**

Components:	Reading lists, guidance notes and MCQ.
Correspondence address:	University Examination Postal Institution Ltd, Mounters Lane, Chawton, Alton, Hants GU34 1RE, UK Tel: 01420–84 184.

Courses for the Part 2 MRCOG

- **Birmingham MRCOG Part 2 Course**

Venue:	Birmingham Women's Hospital, Birmingham.
Dates & Duration:	January / July (1 week).
Components:	Lectures, essays, MCQ and oral assessment.
Correspondence address:	Part 2 MRCOG Course Secretary, Postgraduate Resource Centre, Birmingham Women's Hospital, Birmingham B15 2TG, UK Tel: 0121–472 1377 Ext. 4567.

- **Birmingham MRCOG Part 2 Oral Assessment Course**

Venue:	Birmingham Women's Hospital, Birmingham.
Dates & Duration:	April / October (1 day).
Components:	Lectures, full circuit oral assessment and individual feed back.

Correspondence address: Part 2 MRCOG Course Secretary,
Postgraduate Resource Centre,
Birmingham Women's Hospital,
Birmingham B15 2TG, UK
Tel: 0121–472 1377 Ext. 4567.

• Royal College of Obstetricians & Gynaecologists MRCOG Part 2 Revision Course

Venue:	RCOG, London.
Dates & Duration:	January / July (1 week).
Components:	Lectures, essays, MCQ and oral assessment.
Correspondence address:	Postgraduate Education Department, RCOG, 27 Sussex Place, Regent's Park, London NW1 4RG, UK Tel: 0171–772 6200.

• Whipps Cross Hospital MRCOG Part 2 Revision Course

Venue:	Medical Education Centre, Whipps Cross Hospital, London.
Dates & Duration:	June / November (2 weeks).
Components:	Lectures, essays, MCQ and oral assessment.
Correspondence address:	The Administrator, Medical Education Centre, Whipps Cross Hospital, Whipps Cross Road, Leytonstone, London E11 1NR, UK Tel: 0181–535 6649.

• University of Nottingham MRCOG Part 2 Course

Venue:	Department of Obstetrics & Gynaecology, University of Nottingham.
Dates & Duration:	January / July (2 weeks).
Components:	Lectures, essays, MCQ and oral assessment.
Correspondence address:	Postgraduate Course Co-ordinator, Department of Obstetrics & Gynaecology, University Hospital, Queen's Medical Centre, Nottingham NG7 2UH, UK Tel: 0115–970 9451.

• Queen Charlotte's Hospital Revision Course for MRCOG Part 2

Venue:	Institute of Obstetrics & Gynaecology, Queen Charlotte's & Chelsea Hospital, London.
Dates & Duration:	January / July (2 weeks).
Components:	Lectures (main component), essays, MCQ and oral assessment.
Correspondence address:	Courses Secretary, Institute of Obstetrics & Gynaecology, Queen Charlotte's & Chelsea Hospital, Goldhawk Road, London W6 OXG, UK Tel: 0181–383 3902.

• Queen Charlotte's Hospital Clinical Course for MRCOG Part 2

Venue:	Institute of Obstetrics & Gynaecology, Queen Charlotte's & Chelsea Hospital, London.
Dates & Duration:	April / October (2 weekends).
Components:	Oral assessment.
Correspondence address:	as the previous course.

• Queen Charlotte's Hospital Clinical Study Day for MRCOG Part 2

Venue:	Institute of Obstetrics & Gynaecology, Queen Charlotte's & Chelsea Hospital, London.
Dates & Duration:	April / November (1 day).
Components:	Oral assessment.
Correspondence address:	as the previous course.

• Newcastle MRCOG Part 2 Course

Venue:	Newcastle General Hospital, Newcastle upon Tyne.
Dates & Duration:	June (1 week).
Components:	Lectures, essays, MCQ and oral assessment.

Correspondence address: The Registrar,
Regional Postgraduate Institute of Medicine &
Dentistry,
The University,
11 Framlington Place,
Newcastle upon Tyne NE2 4AB, UK
Tel: 0191–222 6762.

• Edinburgh Postgraduate Board MRCOG Part 2 Theoretical Course

Venue: Lister Postgraduate Institute,
Edinburgh.

Dates & Duration: January / August (1 week).

Components: Lectures, essays and MCQ.

Correspondence address: The Postgraduate Dean,
Edinburgh Postgraduate Board for Medicine,
Pfizer Foundation,
11 Hill Square,
Edinburgh EH8 9DR, UK
Tel: 0131–650 2823.

• Edinburgh Postgraduate Board MRCOG Part 2 Clinical Course

Venue: Royal Infirmary,
Edinburgh.

Dates & Duration: April / October (1 week).

Components: Oral assessment.

Correspondence address: as the previous course.

• University of Keele MRCOG Part 2 Course

Venue: North Staffordshire Hospital Centre,
Stoke-on-Trent.

Dates & Duration: June /December (1 week).

Components: Lectures, essays, MCQ and oral assessment.

Correspondence address: Part 2 MRCOG Course Secretary,
School of Postgraduate Medicine &
Biological Sciences,
Thornburrow Drive,
Hartshill,
Stoke-on-Trent ST4 7QB, UK
Tel: 01782–716 998.

• Liverpool MRCOG Part 2 Course

Venue: Mill Road Maternity Hospital,
                                Liverpool.
Dates & Duration: January / July (1 week).
Components: Essays, MCQ and oral assessment.
Correspondence address: MRCOG Course Secretary,
                                Postgraduate Course Co-ordinator's Office,
                                Mill Road Maternity Hospital,
                                Liverpool L6 2AH, UK
                                Tel: 0151–260 8787 Ext. 2748.

• St George's Hospital MRCOG Part 2 Course

Venue: St George's Hospital Medical School,
                                London.
Dates & Duration: July / October (1 week).
Components: Lectures, essays, MCQ and oral assessment.
Correspondence address: Part 2 MRCOG Course Secretary,
                                Department of Obstetrics & Gynaecology,
                                St George's Hospital Medical School,
                                Cranmer Terrace,
                                London SW17 0RE, UK
                                Tel: 0181–672 9944.

• University of Manchester MRCOG Part 2 Course

Venue: St Mary's Hospital,
                                Manchester.
Dates & Duration: December (2 weeks).
Components: Lectures, essays and MCQ.
                                A weekend of clinical examination practice will
                                be held for those successful in the written
                                examination.
Correspondence address: Courses Administrator,
                                Department of Postgraduate Medical Studies,
                                Gateway House,
                                Piccadilly South
                                Manchester M60 7LP, UK
                                Tel: 0161–237 2714.

• Leeds General Infirmary MRCOG Part 2 Course

Venue:	Clarendon Wing, Leeds General Infirmary, Leeds.
Format:	Two-part revision course.
Dates, Duration & Components:	Part 1 of the Course (January / July): 4 days of lectures, essays and MCQ. Part 2 of the Course (April / October): oral assessment course.
Correspondence address:	Part 2 MRCOG Course Secretary, Academic Unit of Obstetrics and Gynaecology, Clarendon Wing, Leeds General Infirmary, Belmont Grove, Leeds LS2 9NS, UK Tel: 0113–292 3891.

• St James's MRCOG Part 2 Clinical Course

Venue:	Gledhow Wing, St James's University Hospital, Leeds.
Components:	Oral assessment.
Correspondence address:	Part 2 MRCOG Course Secretary, Academic Unit of Obstetrics and Gynaecology, Gledhow Wing, St James's University Hospital, Becket Street, Leeds LS9 7TF, UK Tel: 0113–283 6864.

• Cambridge MRCOG Part 2 Course

Venue:	Rosie Maternity Unit, Addenbrooke's Hospital, Cambridge.
Dates & Duration:	January / July (1 week).
Components:	Lectures, essays, MCQ and oral assessment.
Correspondence address:	Course Secretary, Postgraduate Medical Centre, School of Clinical Medicine, Addenbrooke's Hospital, Cambridge CB2 2SP, UK Tel: 01223–217 105.

• King's College MRCOG Part 2 Theoretical Course

Venue: King's College Hospital,
                                London.
Dates & Duration: January / July (2 weeks).
Components: Lectures, essays and MCQ.
Correspondence address: Course Secretary,
                                Department of Obstetrics & Gynaecology,
                                9th Floor New Ward Block,
                                King's College Hospital,
                                Denmark Hill,
                                London SE5 9RS, UK
                                Tel: 0171–346 3629.

• King's College MRCOG Part 2 Practical Course

Venue: King's College Hospital,
                                London.
Dates & Duration: September / March (4 days).
Components: Oral assessment.
Correspondence address: as the previous course.

• St Thomas' Hospital MRCOG Part 2 Theoretical Course

Venue: St Thomas' Hospital,
                                London.
Dates & Duration: January / July (1 week).
Components: Lectures, essays and MCQ.
Correspondence address: Part 2 MRCOG Course Secretary,
                                Mary Ward,
                                7th Floor, North Wing,
                                St Thomas' Hospital,
                                Lambeth Palace Road,
                                London SE1 7EH, UK
                                Tel: 0171–928 9292.

• St Thomas' Hospital MRCOG Part 2 Clinical Course

Venue: St Thomas' Hospital,
                                London.
Dates & Duration: April / November (1 week).
Components: Oral assessment.
Correspondence address: as the previous course.

• University of Glasgow MRCOG Part 2 Course

Venue:	Glasgow Royal Infirmary, Glasgow.
Dates, Duration & Components:	A split course during the first week of February (lectures, essays and MCQ) and the first week of April (oral assessment).
Correspondence address:	Part 2 MRCOG Course Secretary, Department of Obstetrics & Gynaecology, Royal Infirmary, 10 Alexandra Parade, Glasgow G31 2ER, UK Tel: 0141–552 3535 Ext. 4702.

• University Examination Postal Institution MRCOG Part 2 Correspondence Course

Components:	Reading lists, guidance notes, MCQ and essays marked by a named tutor.
Correspondence address:	University Examination Postal Institution Ltd, Mounters Lane, Chawton, Alton, Hants GU34 1RE, UK Tel: 01420–84184.

Appendix 3

Detailed Instructions and Answer Sheet for the Multiple Choice Question Papers in the Part 1 and the Part 2 MRCOG Examinations

The following instructions have been reproduced with kind permission of Mr Roger Jackson, Examination Secretary, Royal College of Obstetricians and Gynaecologists.

Royal College of Obstetricians and Gynaecologists
27 SUSSEX PLACE, REGENT'S PARK, LONDON NW1 4RG
Telephone: +44 (0) 171-772 6200

Part 1 Membership Examination
Detailed Instructions for the
Multiple Choice Question Paper

This information must be read very carefully. Failure to follow the instructions will result in failure in the examination.

IDENTIFICATION
Candidates must provide evidence of identification, **which includes a photograph,** for inspection prior to commencement of the examination. Candidates failing to provide satisfactory evidence will not be allowed to attend the examination.

THE QUESTION PAPERS
Each paper will consist of sixty (5 part) multiple choice questions in book form. A computer answer sheet will be inserted into the question book and this sheet will be marked by a document reading machine. A sample computer answer sheet is shown overleaf. **You must use only the grade HB pencil provided for completing all parts of the answer sheet.** Pens must not be used for any part of the MCQ examination. Firm pressure is required with the pencil. You must ensure that your marking is bold and dark. You may erase any pencil mark by using the eraser provided.

The time allowed for completion of each MCQ examination is TWO hours. You will be given a warning 30 minutes and 10 minutes before the end of the examination. **Do not start the examinations until instructed by the invigilator.**

FRONT COVER
On the front cover of each question book you must print your full name in the boxes provided and then sign your name in the space marked "signature". Your candidate number (not desk number) must be written in the FOUR SQUARES labelled "CANDIDATE NUMBER".

ANSWER SHEETS (Sample overleaf)
A FIRM DARK IMPRESSION WHICH COMPLETELY FILLS EACH LOZENGE IS ESSENTIAL.
A FAINT LINE WILL NOT BE READ BY THE DOCUMENT READING MACHINE.
The answer sheet must not be folded, creased or torn. You must print your surname (family name) and other name(s) at the top of each answer sheet and write your <u>CANDIDATE NUMBER</u> in the boxes provided. Then **black-out** the lozenges corresponding to your candidate number.

YOU MUST SHOW YOUR NAME AS STATED ON YOUR ENTRY CARD.

QUESTIONS

Each question will consist of an initial statement followed by five items identified by the letters A, B, C, D, E. The answer sheet contains a row of five boxes for each question and is numbered accordingly. Each box refers to a single item. In each box there are two lozenges labelled T(= True) and F(= False). You will be required to indicate whether you know a particular item to be true or false by **boldly** blacking out either the True or False lozenge.

To avoid too many erasures on the answer sheet, candidates may wish to mark their responses in the question book and then transfer their decisions to the answer sheet but this **must** be done **within** the two hours allowed for the examination.

Specimen question and answers

The pudendal nerve:
A. Derives its fibres from the second, third and fourth sacral segments
B. Runs between the pyriformis and coccygeus muscles before leaving the pelvis
C. Has the pudendal artery on its medial side as it lies on the ischial spine
D. Gives off the inferior haemorrhoidal (rectal) nerve in the pudendal canal
E. Innervates the clitoris

Answers A, B, D and E are 'True', answer C is 'False'. Your answer sheet relating to this question would look like this when correctly filled in:

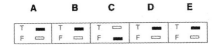

T means TRUE; F means FALSE

MARKING

Each item correctly answered (i.e. a True statement indicated as True or a False statement indicated as False) is awarded one mark (+1). For each incorrect answer no mark (0) is awarded. **All items must be answered true or false. Incorrect answers are not penalised.**

COMPLETION

At the end of each examination insert the completed answer sheet into the question book.

On no account may the question books be removed from the examination hall.

Any candidate who attempts to remove, by writing or by any other means, MCQ examination questions from the examination hall, will be reported to the Examination Committee and will FAIL the whole examination.

Royal College of Obstetricians and Gynaecologists
Part 1 Membership Examination – Paper 1

SURNAME (FAMILY NAME) MARSHALL

OTHER NAME(S) SARAH ELIZABETH

CANDIDATE NUMBER

1 8 5 6

Please use HB pencil. Rub out all errors thoroughly.
Mark lozenges like ▬ NOT like ✓ ✗ ⊖

T = True
F = False

IMPORTANT NOTES

1. When you have finished, check that you have NOT left any blanks.

2. Erasures should be left clean, with no smudges where possible. (The document reading machine will accept the darkest response for each item).

	A	B	C	D	E
1	T F	T F	T F	T F	T F
2	T F	T F	T F	T F	T F
3	T F	T F	T F	T F	T F
4	T F	T F	T F	T F	T F
5	T F	T F	T F	T F	T F
6	T F	T F	T F	T F	T F
7	T F	T F	T F	T F	T F
8	T F	T F	T F	T F	T F
9	T F	T F	T F	T F	T F
10	T F	T F	T F	T F	T F
11	T F	T F	T F	T F	T F
12	T F	T F	T F	T F	T F
13	T F	T F	T F	T F	T F
14	T F	T F	T F	T F	T F
15	T F	T F	T F	T F	T F

	A	B	C	D	E
16	T F	T F	T F	T F	T F
17	T F	T F	T F	T F	T F
18	T F	T F	T F	T F	T F
19	T F	T F	T F	T F	T F
20	T F	T F	T F	T F	T F
21	T F	T F	T F	T F	T F
22	T F	T F	T F	T F	T F
23	T F	T F	T F	T F	T F
24	T F	T F	T F	T F	T F
25	T F	T F	T F	T F	T F
26	T F	T F	T F	T F	T F
27	T F	T F	T F	T F	T F
28	T F	T F	T F	T F	T F
29	T F	T F	T F	T F	T F
30	T F	T F	T F	T F	T F

CHECK THAT YOU HAVE ANSWERED EVERY ITEM TRUE OR FALSE

KENDATA Data Entry Technology   0703 869922

Please use HB pencil. Rub out all errors thoroughly.
Mark lozenges like ▬ NOT like ✔ ✗ ⊝

T = True
F = False

IMPORTANT NOTES

1. When you have finished, check that you have NOT left any blanks.

2. Erasures should be left clean, with no smudges where possible. (The document reading machine will accept the darkest response for each item).

	A	B	C	D	E			A	B	C	D	E
31	T F	T F	T F	T F	T F		**46**	T F	T F	T F	T F	T F
32	T F	T F	T F	T F	T F		**47**	T F	T F	T F	T F	T F
33	T F	T F	T F	T F	T F		**48**	T F	T F	T F	T F	T F
34	T F	T F	T F	T F	T F		**49**	T F	T F	T F	T F	T F
35	T F	T F	T F	T F	T F		**50**	T F	T F	T F	T F	T F
36	T F	T F	T F	T F	T F		**51**	T F	T F	T F	T F	T F
37	T F	T F	T F	T F	T F		**52**	T F	T F	T F	T F	T F
38	T F	T F	T F	T F	T F		**53**	T F	T F	T F	T F	T F
39	T F	T F	T F	T F	T F		**54**	T F	T F	T F	T F	T F
40	T F	T F	T F	T F	T F		**55**	T F	T F	T F	T F	T F
41	T F	T F	T F	T F	T F		**56**	T F	T F	T F	T F	T F
42	T F	T F	T F	T F	T F		**57**	T F	T F	T F	T F	T F
43	T F	T F	T F	T F	T F		**58**	T F	T F	T F	T F	T F
44	T F	T F	T F	T F	T F		**59**	T F	T F	T F	T F	T F
45	T F	T F	T F	T F	T F		**60**	T F	T F	T F	T F	T F

CHECK THAT YOU HAVE ANSWERED EVERY ITEM TRUE OR FALSE

Royal College of Obstetricians and Gynaecologists
27 SUSSEX PLACE, REGENT'S PARK, LONDON NW1 4RG
Telephone : +44 (0) 171-772 6200

Part 2 Membership Examination
Detailed Instructions for the
Multiple Choice Question Paper
in Obstetrics and Gynaecology

This information must be read very carefully. Failure to follow the instructions will result in failure in the examination.

IDENTIFICATION

Candidates must provide, at all sections of the examination evidence of identification, **which must include a photograph,** for inspection prior to commencement of the examination. Candidates failing to provide satisfactory evidence will not be allowed to attend that examination.

THE QUESTION PAPER

The paper will consist of 300 Multiple Choice Questions in book form. A computer Answer Sheet on which answers are to be recorded will be inserted into the Question Book and this sheet will be marked by a document reading machine. A sample computer Answer Sheet is shown overleaf. **You must use only the grade HB pencil provided for completing all parts of the Answer Sheets.** Pens must not be used for any part of the MCQ examination. Firm pressure is required with the pencil. You must ensure that your marking is bold and dark. You may erase any pencil mark by using the eraser provided. The time allowed for completion of the MCQ examination is TWO hours. You will be given a time warning 30 minutes and 10 minutes before the end of the examination. **Do not start the examination until instructed by the invigilator.**

FRONT COVER

On the front cover of each Question Book you must print your full name in the boxes provided and then sign your name in the space marked "signature". Your candidate number (not desk number) must be written in the FOUR SQUARES labelled "CANDIDATE NUMBER".

ANSWER SHEET (Sample overleaf)

A FIRM DARK IMPRESSION WHICH COMPLETELY FILLS EACH LOZENGE IS ESSENTIAL.

A FAINT LINE WILL NOT BE READ BY THE DOCUMENT READING MACHINE.

The Answer Sheet must not be folded, creased or torn. You must print your surname (family name) and other name(s) at the top of the Answer Sheet and write your <u>CANDIDATE NUMBER</u> in the boxes provided. Then **black-out** the lozenges corresponding to your candidate number.

YOU MUST SHOW YOUR NAME AS STATED ON YOUR ENTRY CARD.

ANSWERING THE QUESTIONS

The Answer Sheet is numbered 1-300 and against each number there are two lozenges labelled T(= True) and F(= False). You will be required to indicate whether you know a particular question to be true or false by **boldly** blacking out either the True or False lozenge.

To avoid too many erasures on the Answer Sheet, candidates may wish to mark their responses in the Question Book and then transfer their decisions to the Answer Sheet but this **must** be done **within** the two hours allowed for the examination.

Specimen questions and answers

When compared with radiotherapy, radical hysterectomy
1.   is less favoured in stage 1a carcinoma of the cervix
2.   carries a reduced risk of subsequent lymphocyst formation
3.   allows preservation of ovarian function

Uterine curettage
4.   is associated with an increased incidence of placenta praevia in a subsequent pregnancy
5.   is important in the investigation of secondary infertility

Ovarian Thecomata
6.   are typically benign

The following genital anomalies have a recognised association with the conditions listed:
7.   Hypospadias   :   androgen insensitivity (testicular feminization syndrome)
8.   Hypertrophy
of the clitoris   :   maternal nortestosterone therapy
9.   Varicocele   :   Klinefelter's Syndrome

In a patient with inappropriate lactation associated with secondary amenorrhoea
10.   bitemporal hemianopia on perimetry would be expected in about 25% of patients
11.   an exaggerated rise in serum prolactin concentration following injection of thyrotrophin releasing hormone is a recognised finding
12.   an increased plasma concentration would be expected
13.   treatment with Danazol would be appropriate
14.   the administration of Methyl-Dopa is a recognised cause
15.   anorexia nervosa is a recognised association

Answers 3, 6, 8, 11 and 14 are 'True'; answers 1, 2, 4, 5, 7, 9, 10, 12, 13 and 15 are "False". Your Answer Sheet relating to these questions would look like this when correctly filled in:

MARKING

Each question correctly answered (i.e. a True statement indicated as True or a False statement indicated as False) is awarded one mark (+1). For each incorrect answer no mark (0) is awarded. **All questions must be answered true or false. Incorrect answers are not penalised.**

COMPLETION

At the end of the examination, insert the completed Answer Sheet into the Question Book.

On no account may the Question Book be removed from the examination hall.

Any candidate who attempts to remove, by writing or by any other means, MCQ examination questions from the examination hall, will be reported to the Examination Committee and will FAIL the whole examination.

Royal College of Obstetricians and Gynaecologists
Part 2 Membership Examination

Surname (Family Name)	WILLIAMS		Candidate Number			
			1	9	4	7

Other Name(s)   PETER JOHN

This form will be read by a machine
Please use the HB pencil provided
Mark each answer with a single horizontal line
If you make a mistake erase it completely
Do NOT mark with ticks, crosses or circles
Do not forget to enter your name and candidate number properly

T=True

F=False

IMPORTANT - When you have finished, check that you have answered EVERY question either true or false.
If you leave any question blank it will be scored the same as an incorrect answer.

1 ‹T› ‹F›	31 ‹T› ‹F›	61 ‹T› ‹F›	91 ‹T› ‹F›	121 ‹T› ‹F›
2 ‹T› ‹F›	32 ‹T› ‹F›	62 ‹T› ‹F›	92 ‹T› ‹F›	122 ‹T› ‹F›
3 ‹T› ‹F›	33 ‹T› ‹F›	63 ‹T› ‹F›	93 ‹T› ‹F›	123 ‹T› ‹F›
4 ‹T› ‹F›	34 ‹T› ‹F›	64 ‹T› ‹F›	94 ‹T› ‹F›	124 ‹T› ‹F›
5 ‹T› ‹F›	35 ‹T› ‹F›	65 ‹T› ‹F›	95 ‹T› ‹F›	125 ‹T› ‹F›
6 ‹T› ‹F›	36 ‹T› ‹F›	66 ‹T› ‹F›	96 ‹T› ‹F›	126 ‹T› ‹F›
7 ‹T› ‹F›	37 ‹T› ‹F›	67 ‹T› ‹F›	97 ‹T› ‹F›	127 ‹T› ‹F›
8 ‹T› ‹F›	38 ‹T› ‹F›	68 ‹T› ‹F›	98 ‹T› ‹F›	128 ‹T› ‹F›
9 ‹T› ‹F›	39 ‹T› ‹F›	69 ‹T› ‹F›	99 ‹T› ‹F›	129 ‹T› ‹F›
10 ‹T› ‹F›	40 ‹T› ‹F›	70 ‹T› ‹F›	100 ‹T› ‹F›	130 ‹T› ‹F›
11 ‹T› ‹F›	41 ‹T› ‹F›	71 ‹T› ‹F›	101 ‹T› ‹F›	131 ‹T› ‹F›
12 ‹T› ‹F›	42 ‹T› ‹F›	72 ‹T› ‹F›	102 ‹T› ‹F›	132 ‹T› ‹F›
13 ‹T› ‹F›	43 ‹T› ‹F›	73 ‹T› ‹F›	103 ‹T› ‹F›	133 ‹T› ‹F›
14 ‹T› ‹F›	44 ‹T› ‹F›	74 ‹T› ‹F›	104 ‹T› ‹F›	134 ‹T› ‹F›
15 ‹T› ‹F›	45 ‹T› ‹F›	75 ‹T› ‹F›	105 ‹T› ‹F›	135 ‹T› ‹F›
16 ‹T› ‹F›	46 ‹T› ‹F›	76 ‹T› ‹F›	106 ‹T› ‹F›	136 ‹T› ‹F›
17 ‹T› ‹F›	47 ‹T› ‹F›	77 ‹T› ‹F›	107 ‹T› ‹F›	137 ‹T› ‹F›
18 ‹T› ‹F›	48 ‹T› ‹F›	78 ‹T› ‹F›	108 ‹T› ‹F›	138 ‹T› ‹F›
19 ‹T› ‹F›	49 ‹T› ‹F›	79 ‹T› ‹F›	109 ‹T› ‹F›	139 ‹T› ‹F›
20 ‹T› ‹F›	50 ‹T› ‹F›	80 ‹T› ‹F›	110 ‹T› ‹F›	140 ‹T› ‹F›
21 ‹T› ‹F›	51 ‹T› ‹F›	81 ‹T› ‹F›	111 ‹T› ‹F›	141 ‹T› ‹F›
22 ‹T› ‹F›	52 ‹T› ‹F›	82 ‹T› ‹F›	112 ‹T› ‹F›	142 ‹T› ‹F›
23 ‹T› ‹F›	53 ‹T› ‹F›	83 ‹T› ‹F›	113 ‹T› ‹F›	143 ‹T› ‹F›
24 ‹T› ‹F›	54 ‹T› ‹F›	84 ‹T› ‹F›	114 ‹T› ‹F›	144 ‹T› ‹F›
25 ‹T› ‹F›	55 ‹T› ‹F›	85 ‹T› ‹F›	115 ‹T› ‹F›	145 ‹T› ‹F›
26 ‹T› ‹F›	56 ‹T› ‹F›	86 ‹T› ‹F›	116 ‹T› ‹F›	146 ‹T› ‹F›
27 ‹T› ‹F›	57 ‹T› ‹F›	87 ‹T› ‹F›	117 ‹T› ‹F›	147 ‹T› ‹F›
28 ‹T› ‹F›	58 ‹T› ‹F›	88 ‹T› ‹F›	118 ‹T› ‹F›	148 ‹T› ‹F›
29 ‹T› ‹F›	59 ‹T› ‹F›	89 ‹T› ‹F›	119 ‹T› ‹F›	149 ‹T› ‹F›
30 ‹T› ‹F›	60 ‹T› ‹F›	90 ‹T› ‹F›	120 ‹T› ‹F›	150 ‹T› ‹F›

Check that you have answered every question either True or False.

This form will be read by a machine
Please use the HB pencil provided
Mark each answer with a single horizontal line
If you make a mistake erase it completely
Do NOT mark with ticks, crosses or circles
Do not forget to enter your name and candidate number properly

T=True

F=False

IMPORTANT - When you have finished, check that you have answered EVERY question either true or false.
If you leave any question blank it will be scored the same as an incorrect answer.

151 ⟨T⟩ ⟨F⟩	181 ⟨T⟩ ⟨F⟩	211 ⟨T⟩ ⟨F⟩	241 ⟨T⟩ ⟨F⟩	271 ⟨T⟩ ⟨F⟩
152 ⟨T⟩ ⟨F⟩	182 ⟨T⟩ ⟨F⟩	212 ⟨T⟩ ⟨F⟩	242 ⟨T⟩ ⟨F⟩	272 ⟨T⟩ ⟨F⟩
153 ⟨T⟩ ⟨F⟩	183 ⟨T⟩ ⟨F⟩	213 ⟨T⟩ ⟨F⟩	243 ⟨T⟩ ⟨F⟩	273 ⟨T⟩ ⟨F⟩
154 ⟨T⟩ ⟨F⟩	184 ⟨T⟩ ⟨F⟩	214 ⟨T⟩ ⟨F⟩	244 ⟨T⟩ ⟨F⟩	274 ⟨T⟩ ⟨F⟩
155 ⟨T⟩ ⟨F⟩	185 ⟨T⟩ ⟨F⟩	215 ⟨T⟩ ⟨F⟩	245 ⟨T⟩ ⟨F⟩	275 ⟨T⟩ ⟨F⟩
156 ⟨T⟩ ⟨F⟩	186 ⟨T⟩ ⟨F⟩	216 ⟨T⟩ ⟨F⟩	246 ⟨T⟩ ⟨F⟩	276 ⟨T⟩ ⟨F⟩
157 ⟨T⟩ ⟨F⟩	187 ⟨T⟩ ⟨F⟩	217 ⟨T⟩ ⟨F⟩	247 ⟨T⟩ ⟨F⟩	277 ⟨T⟩ ⟨F⟩
158 ⟨T⟩ ⟨F⟩	188 ⟨T⟩ ⟨F⟩	218 ⟨T⟩ ⟨F⟩	248 ⟨T⟩ ⟨F⟩	278 ⟨T⟩ ⟨F⟩
159 ⟨T⟩ ⟨F⟩	189 ⟨T⟩ ⟨F⟩	219 ⟨T⟩ ⟨F⟩	249 ⟨T⟩ ⟨F⟩	279 ⟨T⟩ ⟨F⟩
160 ⟨T⟩ ⟨F⟩	190 ⟨T⟩ ⟨F⟩	220 ⟨T⟩ ⟨F⟩	250 ⟨T⟩ ⟨F⟩	280 ⟨T⟩ ⟨F⟩
161 ⟨T⟩ ⟨F⟩	191 ⟨T⟩ ⟨F⟩	221 ⟨T⟩ ⟨F⟩	251 ⟨T⟩ ⟨F⟩	281 ⟨T⟩ ⟨F⟩
162 ⟨T⟩ ⟨F⟩	192 ⟨T⟩ ⟨F⟩	222 ⟨T⟩ ⟨F⟩	252 ⟨T⟩ ⟨F⟩	282 ⟨T⟩ ⟨F⟩
163 ⟨T⟩ ⟨F⟩	193 ⟨T⟩ ⟨F⟩	223 ⟨T⟩ ⟨F⟩	253 ⟨T⟩ ⟨F⟩	283 ⟨T⟩ ⟨F⟩
164 ⟨T⟩ ⟨F⟩	194 ⟨T⟩ ⟨F⟩	224 ⟨T⟩ ⟨F⟩	254 ⟨T⟩ ⟨F⟩	284 ⟨T⟩ ⟨F⟩
165 ⟨T⟩ ⟨F⟩	195 ⟨T⟩ ⟨F⟩	225 ⟨T⟩ ⟨F⟩	255 ⟨T⟩ ⟨F⟩	285 ⟨T⟩ ⟨F⟩
166 ⟨T⟩ ⟨F⟩	196 ⟨T⟩ ⟨F⟩	226 ⟨T⟩ ⟨F⟩	256 ⟨T⟩ ⟨F⟩	286 ⟨T⟩ ⟨F⟩
167 ⟨T⟩ ⟨F⟩	197 ⟨T⟩ ⟨F⟩	227 ⟨T⟩ ⟨F⟩	257 ⟨T⟩ ⟨F⟩	287 ⟨T⟩ ⟨F⟩
168 ⟨T⟩ ⟨F⟩	198 ⟨T⟩ ⟨F⟩	228 ⟨T⟩ ⟨F⟩	258 ⟨T⟩ ⟨F⟩	288 ⟨T⟩ ⟨F⟩
169 ⟨T⟩ ⟨F⟩	199 ⟨T⟩ ⟨F⟩	229 ⟨T⟩ ⟨F⟩	259 ⟨T⟩ ⟨F⟩	289 ⟨T⟩ ⟨F⟩
170 ⟨T⟩ ⟨F⟩	200 ⟨T⟩ ⟨F⟩	230 ⟨T⟩ ⟨F⟩	260 ⟨T⟩ ⟨F⟩	290 ⟨T⟩ ⟨F⟩
171 ⟨T⟩ ⟨F⟩	201 ⟨T⟩ ⟨F⟩	231 ⟨T⟩ ⟨F⟩	261 ⟨T⟩ ⟨F⟩	291 ⟨T⟩ ⟨F⟩
172 ⟨T⟩ ⟨F⟩	202 ⟨T⟩ ⟨F⟩	232 ⟨T⟩ ⟨F⟩	262 ⟨T⟩ ⟨F⟩	292 ⟨T⟩ ⟨F⟩
173 ⟨T⟩ ⟨F⟩	203 ⟨T⟩ ⟨F⟩	233 ⟨T⟩ ⟨F⟩	263 ⟨T⟩ ⟨F⟩	293 ⟨T⟩ ⟨F⟩
174 ⟨T⟩ ⟨F⟩	204 ⟨T⟩ ⟨F⟩	234 ⟨T⟩ ⟨F⟩	264 ⟨T⟩ ⟨F⟩	294 ⟨T⟩ ⟨F⟩
175 ⟨T⟩ ⟨F⟩	205 ⟨T⟩ ⟨F⟩	235 ⟨T⟩ ⟨F⟩	265 ⟨T⟩ ⟨F⟩	295 ⟨T⟩ ⟨F⟩
176 ⟨T⟩ ⟨F⟩	206 ⟨T⟩ ⟨F⟩	236 ⟨T⟩ ⟨F⟩	266 ⟨T⟩ ⟨F⟩	296 ⟨T⟩ ⟨F⟩
177 ⟨T⟩ ⟨F⟩	207 ⟨T⟩ ⟨F⟩	237 ⟨T⟩ ⟨F⟩	267 ⟨T⟩ ⟨F⟩	297 ⟨T⟩ ⟨F⟩
178 ⟨T⟩ ⟨F⟩	208 ⟨T⟩ ⟨F⟩	238 ⟨T⟩ ⟨F⟩	268 ⟨T⟩ ⟨F⟩	298 ⟨T⟩ ⟨F⟩
179 ⟨T⟩ ⟨F⟩	209 ⟨T⟩ ⟨F⟩	239 ⟨T⟩ ⟨F⟩	269 ⟨T⟩ ⟨F⟩	299 ⟨T⟩ ⟨F⟩
180 ⟨T⟩ ⟨F⟩	210 ⟨T⟩ ⟨F⟩	240 ⟨T⟩ ⟨F⟩	270 ⟨T⟩ ⟨F⟩	300 ⟨T⟩ ⟨F⟩

Check that you have answered every question either True or False.

System Design by Speedwell Computing Services. 01604 410041   Mark Reflex® by NCSi NM-01317:654321   ED3803   Printed in the U.K.

Paper 2 page 4

Index